Vascular Neurosurgery

Samer S. Hoz

Vascular Neurosurgery

In Multiple-Choice Questions

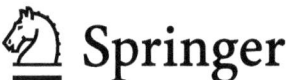 Springer

Samer S. Hoz
Neurosurgery Teaching Hospital
Baghdad, Iraq

ISBN 978-3-319-49186-8   ISBN 978-3-319-49187-5   (eBook)
DOI 10.1007/978-3-319-49187-5

Library of Congress Control Number: 2017934338

Printed on acid-free paper

This Springer imprint is published by Springer Nature
The registered company is Springer International Publishing AG
The registered company address is: Gewerbestrasse 11, 6330 Cham, Switzerland

To the founders of neurological surgery in IRAQ:
Dr. Saad H. Al-Witry
Dr. Tariq Abdul-Wahid
Dr. Sameer H. Aboud
Dr. Rafid Al-Saffar
Dr. Hikmat Sideeq
Dr. A Hadi Al Khalili
Dr. Imad Hashim Ahmad
Dr. Ari Sami H. Nadhim
To my respectful teacher and mentor:
Dr. Anwer Noori Hafidh
To my lovely family:
Mom: Sawsan
Dad: Saad
Sister: Samher
Wife: Arwa
Daughters: Farah and Ward

Foreword by Peter Nakaji

Cerebrovascular surgery is among the most challenging of the disciplines in neurosurgery. Its stakes are high and the field is complex and experiencing a high rate of evolution. Neurosurgeons who choose to face its challenges must constantly perfect their knowledge and skills to be equal to its formidable tasks. One of the best ways to stay current is to test oneself. You hold in your hands a most compelling instrument to achieve that aim.

This volume by Dr. Hoz and his colleagues represents a study tool that covers the key content areas of vascular neurosurgery. The student of neurosurgery, the resident, the fellow, and the younger neurosurgeon preparing for board exams or practice will be the most obvious beneficiaries from this work.

The question and answer format is accessible, direct, and time efficient. I believe it is one of the most valuable forms of study. The answers in this guide are detailed yet clearly are distillations of the most important information, from which the extraneous have been wisely excluded.

One recalls the famous quote of Antoine de Saint-Exupéry that perfection is attained not when there is no longer more to add but when there is no longer anything to take away. The reader would do well to read this well-chosen content even if he or she gets the answer correct, as there is much to be gained from its review. Even later stage neurosurgeons can benefit from the effort to go through it, as I have myself.

We would all be remiss not to recognize a remarkable feature of this book. Dr. Hoz is a neurosurgery resident in Baghdad, Iraq, who made the effort to envision and edit this book. I have not been to Baghdad, but I feel confident in speculating that it is not the easiest place in the world to practice complex cerebrovascular neurosurgery. However, I do not doubt that the clinical problems facing humans there are the same as anywhere.

I met Dr. Hoz when he came to one of our bypass courses at the Barrow Neurological Institute. He is clearly passionate about vascular neurosurgery and dedicated to improving himself so he can bring his patients the highest level of care. On the one hand, his book shows that the same key information in vascular neurosurgery is true and relevant the world over; on the other, it reminds us that no amount of turbulence or adversity in our environment should allay us from our responsibility to learn and share learning for the benefit of our patients and the field.

I recommend this volume to you and hope you will make it a living part of your library. I have no doubt you will find it as useful as I have—and you may be delighted to find some unexpected extra dewdrops of inspiration and passion for vascular neurosurgery that its editor in his labors left within.

Peter Nakaji, MD
Division of Neurological Surgery
Barrow Neurological Institute
Phoenix, AZ, USA

Executive Committee of Congress of Neurological Surgery
Schaumburg, IL, USA

Foreword by Suresh M. Dugani

Dear Dr. Samer Hoz,

Thank you very much for considering me for the opinion and suggestions for your excellent book on *vascular neurosurgery* multiple-choice questions, explanations, and answers; indeed, it is pleasure and honor for me.

I went through the whole book and every question and choices and answers in detail. As I was going through, I could not put it down till the end. It is highly scientific, educative, and informative. I felt there is extensive work and effort put in preparing this book.

All the topics as basics anatomy, physiology, clinical aspects, diagnosis and management of every neurovascular problems is addressed with comprehensive information.

As a professor and consultant, finer details in neurovascular surgery I came to know, after going through the book. It delivers comprehensive information on neurovascular surgical speciality in the form of intricate, finer questions, explanations and answers.

I am sure, it will be wonderful teaching, learning material to all neurosciences, residents, trainees, faculty and consultants.

I heartily thank and congratulate Dr. Samer Hoz for this excellent work and wish he keeps it up with newer editions and contributes for the growth and development of neurosciences, and I wish him all the best.

Suresh M. Dugani
Department of Neurosurgery
S.D.M. Medical College
Dharwad, Karnataka, India

Regional Neurosciences Centre
Shiva Krupa Hospital
Hubli-Dharwad, Karnataka, India

Foreword by Roberto R. Herrera

When author Dr. Samer S. Hoz asked me to do a foreword to his book, I felt a great responsibility. After reading and analyzing the text, I can say today that it is my pleasure and my honor to write this foreword to the book *Vascular Neurosurgery: In Multiple-Choice Questions*. This is an exceptional work that covers all aspects of modern vascular neurosurgery from the brain to the spinal cord, covering the clinical aspects, diagnosis, and treatment.

The questions and choices are made in a succinct, practical, and concrete way, facilitating the analysis and study of the answers.

This book will be useful mainly for young neurosurgeons around the world, residents, trainers, and students, and how it was conceived will also help experienced neurosurgeons, neurologists, and specialists in neurological intensive care.

Thanks to the author for considering me to give my opinion about his book. I want to congratulate him and wish him the best on the publication of this work and hope that the future edition reaches the success that Dr. Hoz and his colleagues deserve.

Roberto R. Herrera
Neurosurgical Department
Director Intraoperative Magnetic Resonance Imaging Program
Belgrano Adventist Clinic
Buenos Aires, Argentina

Foreword by Renato J. Galzio

Vascular Neurosurgery represents, as well stated in the title, a study companion guide especially directed to residents and young neurosurgeons, but also of considerable interest for the more expert ones.

This book focuses on vascular pathologies of neurosurgical relevance, using an alternative format based on questions with multiple answers. It doesn't replace classical neurosurgical manuals and books but rather may act as a stimulus to learn more and to encourage discussion about this kind of complex diseases.

It is an optimal educational tool, also providing a number of bibliographic references, useful to extend in the deep the study of these topics.

Renato J. Galzio, MD
Department of Life, Health & Environmental Sciences
Division of Neurosurgery
University of L'Aquila
L'Aquila, Italy

Operative Unit of Neurosurgery
San Salvatore City Hospital
L'Aquila, Italy

Foreword by Iype Cherian

As one travels more and more among the vascular system of the brain, the respect and the awe that one has for this amazing network of vessels increases. One realizes that the "tree of life" inside the brain along with the paravascular pathways helps the huge supercomputer called the brain to sustain and work.

The anomalies of the vascular system are varied and many, as has been highlighted in this book, and we, as vascular surgeons, have been doing the "plumbing job" without much understanding of "what really lies beneath." Endovascular surgery has progressed in a spectacular fashion, and most of us, surviving vascular surgeons, might hold on to the "surgery is better" dictum, at least till we retire. And maybe in trained hands, it is the truth to some extent, as well. However, time will tell what is better. It always does.

In an era where acquiring neurosurgical skills is secondary to writing papers, I am sure that this book would throw sparks of interest into the young neurosurgeons' minds about a science which has a realm way above our plumbing jobs, open or closed. As they say in the olden times, "Asathoma sat gamaya, thamasoma jyothir gamaya, mruthyoma amrutham gamaya" which has the following meaning, "From the untruth lead us to the truth, from the darkness lead us to light, and from being dead lead us to life."

This book is a great addition to residents and junior and senior neurosurgeons engaged in the vascular surgery field. My best wishes to SAMER and his team for this spectacular effort from Iraq. Being in Nepal for the last 10 years makes me understand to an extent how hard this team would have worked to put this book together. I would also like to wish all my best to his future endeavors.

Iype Cherian
Department of Neurosurgery
COMS, Bharatpur, Nepal

Counselor, Asian Congress of Neurological Surgeons
Member, WFNS anatomy committee
Bharatpur, Nepal

Preface

A physician who seeks the most challenging aspect of the field is the neurosurgeon. That is my definition of our specialty, which deals with the most eloquent organs in the body (the brain and the spinal cord) that are unique in everything such as lacking significant regeneration and perceptible healing process to the original normal status.

If you consider the above, the vascular neurosurgery will represent the extreme example of challenge within the field of neurosurgery. A highly demanding project requires not only extraordinary surgical skills and orientation from the vascular neurosurgeon but requires an interactive team of neuroradiology, neuro-anesthesia, neurointensive care, neurophysiology, neurology, neuropathology, and neuro-paramedics all with an ultimate dedication.

During the third year of my neurosurgery residency, I decided to go as extreme as possible to be a vascular neurosurgeon in the future. This is unexpected to be an easygoing process, especially in Iraq where the subspecialties in the field are not even accepted idea until now. Therefore, you must build an acceptance of the subspecialty idea within the field of neurosurgery first, and that will be unlikely without "out of the box" steps to enhance such hope. Here, the idea of writing a book in the vascular specialty with consolidated scientific contents and strong correlation and support from international pioneers in the field and a trust-worthy giant publisher came to be the promising step that must be proved before proceeding to the next era.

I put this humble book to be a guide to the mysterious vascular aspect of neurosurgery, trying to concentrate on the core, intended to help the reader via a systematic approach to diagnose and manage the common vascular neurosurgical problems using the art of applying scientific knowledge to practice.

It is the FIRST review book to use the multiple-choice question format in vascular neurosurgery, and it contains over 330 questions and all are genuine (new). These questions are designed to provide a refresher course either in long or briefer study sessions as time permits during a busy day on the neurosurgical practice.

This book is an adjuvant to the present texts and does not intent to be a sole source of knowledge but target the candidate's strengths and identify areas of potential weakness. Constructive commentary is always welcome. I hope that you enjoy reading this book as much as I did putting it together. Good luck!

Samer S. Hoz
Baghdad, Iraq

Acknowledgments

The editor would like to thank the following individuals for their assistance and contributions to this project: *Dr. Osama Al-Awadi* (president of Iraqi Association of Neurosurgeons), *Dr. Ali K. Alshalchy* (college of medicine. Baghdad university: dean), *Dr. Moneer K. faraj* (Arabic board of Neurosurgery: chairman), *DR. Abdulameer Jasim* (of Iraqi board of Neurosurgery: chairman), *Dr. Ahmad Adnan Al-Juboury, Dr. Mohammed A. Mousa, Dr. Mohammed Abdullah, Dr. Hayder Salih, Dr. Wisam Hussein, Dr. Saif Saood, Dr. Mohammed Sabah, Dr. Mohammed Ameen, Dr. Ibrahim Allawi, Dr. Hayder Ali Ammar, Dr. Sarmad Najat, Dr. Alhassan Alnsairy, Dr. Maher Khashea, Dr. Mohammed Burhan* and *Dr. Aysar Khudhair.*

The editor also has a lot of appreciation and gratitude to the supporting seniors and colleagues in the neurosurgery teaching hospital in Baghdad, Iraq: the seniors, *Dr. Yaqthan Al-Azawi, Dr. Ahmad Amman, Dr. Jasem Mohammed, Dr. Ahmed Radhi Obaid, Dr. Sadik Fadhel, Dr. Haider Tawfeeq, Dr. Kadhum Al-Khozaai, Dr. Waleed Al-Hayali, Dr. Raad Sajed, Dr. Basim Nema, Dr. Riyadh Ahmed, Dr. Zaki Ibrahem, Dr. Sameer Hameed,* and *Dr. Ziad Tariq,* and the colleagues, *Dr. Mustafa Hameed, Dr. Salman Ahmad, Dr. Haider Faris, Dr. Ali Saood,* and *Dr. Hassan Zuhair.*

About This Book

— *Vascular Neurosurgery* is the *first guide* dedicated to bring the light to the mysterious world of vascular pathologies affecting the central nervous system.

— *Vascular Neurosurgery* mission is to help readers comprehend the material and retain this knowledge, rather than solely striving for the answer in tricky way.

— This essential review mirrors the exam's multiple-choice format, and the *seven chapters* provide comprehensive coverage of the core concepts in vascular neurosurgery.

— This study companion offers *349 MCQs* in a convenient format that is ideal for self-study, and all the MCQs are *genuine* (all MCQs are new and not adopted from other question books).

— The plan and structure of the questions give a *stepwise comprehensive description* of each disease from the definition, related anatomy, pathology, clinical features, radiology to the surgical decision, and operative tricks, giving an enjoyable and concise review.

— Answers and explanations appear *directly below the questions* to enable easy reading on the go.

— *Vascular Neurosurgery* is essential review for residents across neurosurgical disciplines and contains most of the neurovascular informations the neurosurgical residents need to prepare for their certification exam. It is also beneficial for those seeking a refresher or for those preparing for maintenance of certification.

This book contains some difficult questions marked with "*" sign.

Contents

About the Author

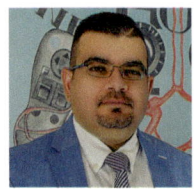

Samer Saad Hoz
Graduated from college of medicine, Baghdad-University 2006. Resident of neurological surgery in the Neurosurgery Teaching Hospital, Baghdad Iraq. Interested in vascular neurosurgery. Director of the first neurosurgery skills training lab in Iraq. Conducting several academic presentations at international conferences. Working on several academic researches under publishing.

Abbreviations

ACA A1, A2, A3, A4, or A5	Anterior cerebral artery	CMs	Cavernous malformations or cavernomas
	Anterior cerebral artery (parts)	CN	Cranial nerve
		CNS	Central nervous system
AChA	Anterior choroidal artery	CS	Cavernous sinus
ACP	Anterior clinoid process	CSF	Cerebrospinal fluid
Acom	Anterior communicating artery	CT	Computed tomography
		CTA	Computed tomography angiography
ADPKD	Autosomal dominant polycystic kidney disease	DACA	Distal anterior cerebral artery aneurysms
ADPLD	Autosomal dominant polycystic liver disease	DAVFs	Dural arteriovenous fistulas
AICA	Anterior inferior cerebellar artery	DSA	Digital subtraction angiography
AKA	Also known as	DVA	Developmental venous anomaly
AOVMs	Angiographically occult (or cryptic) vascular malformations		
ASA	Anterior spinal artery	EC-IC	External carotid-internal carotid
AV shunt	Arteriovenous shunt	ECA	External carotid artery
AVF	Arteriovenous fistula	ED	Extradural
AVMs	Arteriovenous malformations	EDAMS	Encephalo-duro-arterio-myo-synangiosis
		EDH	Extradural hematoma
BB	Basilar bifurcation	EEG	Electroencephalography
BTAs	Basilar trunk aneurysms	EMS	Encephalo-myo-synangiosis
BTO	Balloon test occlusion	EVD	External ventricular drain
CA	Carcinoma	FA	Fusiform aneurysm
CBF	Cerebral blood flow	FIO2	Fractional inspired oxygen
CCF	Carotid-cavernous fistula		
CHF	Congestive heart failure	FLAIR	Fluid attenuation inversion recovery
CISS	Constructive interference in steady state		
CMA	Callosomarginal artery	GE	Gradient echo

ICA	Internal carotid artery	PCP	Posterior clinoid process
ICB aneurysms	Internal carotid artery bifurcation aneurysms	PET	Positron emission tomography
ICH	Intracerebral hematoma	PICA	Posterior inferior cerebellar artery
ICP	Intracranial pressure	PSA	Posterior spinal artery
ID	Intradural		
ISUIA	International Study of Unruptured Intracranial Aneurysms	RAH	Recurrent artery of Heubner
IVH	Intraventricular hemorrhage	SAH	Subarachnoid hemorrhage
		SAS	Subarachnoid Space
MC	Most common	SAVMs	Spinal arteriovenous malformations
MCA	Middle cerebral artery	SCA	Superior cerebral artery
M1, M2, M3, M4, or M5	Middle cerebral artery (parts)	SDH	Subdural hematoma
		SOF	Superior orbital fissure
MMD	Moyamoya disease	SPECT	Single photon emission computed tomography
MRA	Magnetic resonance imaging	STA	Superficial temporal artery
		STG	Superior temporal gyrus
NF	Neurofibromatosis		
		T1WI	T1-weighted image
Op	Operation	T2WI	T2-weighted image
OphA	Ophthalmic artery	TIA	Transient ischemic attack
OS	Optic strut	TICAs	Traumatic intracranial aneurysms
OZ	Orbitozygomatic		
		TVE	Transvenous embolization
PAVEL	Pterional approach via the extended lateral corridor	USG	Ultrasonography
PCA	Posterior cerebral artery	V1 or V2 or V2	Fifth cranial nerve (trigeminal nerve) divisions
P1, P2, P3, P4, or P5	Posterior cerebral artery (parts)		
Pcom	Posterior communicating artery	VA	Vertebral artery
		VBJ	Vertebrobasilar junction

Abbreviations

VGAD Vein of Galen aneurysmal dilation

VGAMs Vein of Galen aneurysmal malformations

VGV Vein of Galen varix

WFNS World Federation of Neurological Surgery

3D CTA Three-dimensional computed tomography angiography

Intracranial Aneurysms

This book contains some difficult questions marked with " * " sign.

© Springer International Publishing AG 2017
S.S. Hoz, *Vascular Neurosurgery*, DOI 10.1007/978-3-319-49187-5_1

? 1. Intracranial aneurysms
   General, the FALSE answer is:
   A. Intracranial aneurysms affect 5–10 % of the general population.
   B. The Acom region is the most common site for intracranial aneurysms.
   C. ICA is the second most common location.
   D. MCA is more common than ICA location.
   E. Ratio of ruptured: unruptured intracranial aneurysms is about 50 %.

✓ The answer is **D.**
   ▬ ICA is the second most common location, while MCA is the third most common location.
   ▬ Intracranial aneurysms affect 5–10 % of the general population.
   ▬ The Acom region is the most common site for intracranial aneurysms. However, aneurysms in this location can be missed on angiography.
   ▬ Ratio of ruptured: unruptured (incidental) aneurysm is 5:3–5:6 (rough estimate is 1:1).

? 2. Intracranial aneurysms
   General (anterior circulation), the FALSE answer is:
   A. Incidence of Acom-ACA aneurysms is 39 %.
   B. Incidence of Pcom aneurysms is 25 %.
   C. Incidence of MCA aneurysms is 20 %.
   D. Incidence of DACA is 6 %.
   E. MCA aneurysms usually at the M3/M4 junction.

✓ The answer is **E.**
   ▬ Incidence of MCA aneurysms (usually at the M1/M2 junction) is 20 %.

? 3. Intracranial aneurysms
   General (posterior circulation), the FALSE answer is:
   A. Approximately 15 % of saccular aneurysms occur in the vertebro-basilar system.
   B. Dissections and fusiform aneurysms are more common in the posterior than in the anterior circulation.
   C. Posterior circulation aneurysms occur most often at the basilar tip followed by the origins of SCA and PICA.
   D. Basilar tip aneurysms account for 50 % of posterior circulation aneurysms.
   E. Vertebral artery aneurysms account for 5 % of posterior circulation aneurysms.

✅ The answer is **E**.
- ― VA aneurysms account for 5 % of all intracranial aneurysms.
- ― VA-PICA junction is the most common site in vertebral artery aneurysms.

❓ 4. **Intracranial aneurysms**
General, the FALSE answer is:
A. Incidence of pediatric intracranial aneurysms is 20 %.
B. Incidence of multiple aneurysms is 15–20 %.
C. Incidence of giant aneurysms is 2–5 %.
D. Incidence of infectious intracranial aneurysms is 2–5 %.
E. Incidence of traumatic intracranial aneurysms is 1 %.

✅ The answer is **A**.
- ― Only 2 % of aneurysms present during childhood.

❓ 5. **Intracranial aneurysms**
General, the FALSE answer is:
A. Acom complex is the commonest location for ruptured aneurysms.
B. Acom complex is also the commonest for coincidental and unruptured aneurysms.
C. Unusual aneurysm locations should alert one to possible unusual causes like infection.
D. Medially directed carotid cavernous aneurysm may be the result of arterial damage during paranasal sinus surgery or hypophysectomy.
E. Distal vertebral fusiform aneurysms are likely to be due to dissection.

✅ The answer is **B**.
- ― MCA is the commonest for coincidental and unruptured aneurysms.

❓ 6. **Intracranial aneurysms**
General rules of aneurysm formation, the FALSE answer is:
A. Aneurysms arise at a branching site on the parent artery.
B. Fusiform aneurysms arise at a turn or curve in the artery.
C. The aneurysm dome or fundus points in the direction of the maximal hemodynamic thrust.
D. There is a constantly occurring set of perforating arteries situated at each aneurysm site that need to be protected and preserved.
E. Most of the persistent carotid-basilar anastomoses have been reported to be associated with aneurysms and SAH.

✅ The answer is **B**.
- Saccular aneurysms arise at a turn or curve in the artery.
- In 1979, Rhoton introduced three rules related to the anatomy of saccular aneurysms that should be considered when planning the operative approach to these lesions.
- First, these aneurysms arise at a branching site on the parent artery. This site may be formed either by the origin of a side branch from the parent artery, such as the origin of the Pcom from the ICA, or by subdivision of a main arterial trunk into two trunks, as occurs at the bifurcation of the middle cerebral or basilar arteries.
- Second, saccular aneurysms arise at a turn or curve in the artery. These curves, by producing local alterations in intravascular hemodynamics, exert unusual stresses on apical regions that receive the greatest force of the pulse wave. Saccular aneurysms arise on the convex, not concave, side of the curve.
- Third, saccular aneurysms point in the direction that the blood would have gone if the curve at the aneurysm site were not present. The aneurysm dome or fundus points in the direction of the maximal hemodynamic thrust in the pre-aneurysmal segment of the parent artery.
- Since the original introduction of the three rules, new anatomic studies have revealed a fourth rule. The fourth rule is that there is a constantly occurring set of perforating arteries situated at each aneurysm site that need to be protected and preserved to achieve an optimal result.
- A fifth rule was added which state that all of the persistent carotid-basilar anastomoses have been reported in association with aneurysms and SAH, including the trigeminal, hypoglossal, otic, and proatlantal arteries.

❓ 7. **Intracranial aneurysms***
   General relevant anatomy (anomalies of ACA), the FALSE answer is:
   A. Type I anomaly: azygous (single) ACA is rare.
   B. Type III anomaly is the most common type.
   C. Type III anomaly includes unpaired ACA.
   D. The A1 segments are equal in size in only 19 %.
   E. Not infrequently, a hypoplastic A1 segment is associated with a large Acom.

✅ The answer is **C**.
Anomalies of ACA are common, especially in patients with aneurysms.
- Azygous ACA, the "unpaired ACA" (**type I** anomaly) is rare.
- **Type II** anomaly is "bihemispheric ACA" as an A2 segment of the ACA that sends branches across the midline to both hemispheres, usually in the presence of a contralateral A2 segment that is either hypoplastic or that terminates early in its course toward the genu of the corpus callosum.

- The most common (**type III** anomaly) is the "accessory ACA," defined as a third artery originating from the Acom, in addition to the paired A2, usually in the midline and with branches to one or both hemispheres.
- Not infrequently, a hypoplastic A1 segment is associated with a large Acom, and aneurysms arise from the side of the large ACA in over 95 %.

❓ 8. Intracranial aneurysms
General relevant anatomy, the FALSE answer is:
   A. The recurrent artery of Heubner runs parallel to the A2.
   B. The recurrent artery of Heubner usually arises from A2 segment in about 90 % of patients.
   C. Pcom is hypoplastic in about 10 % of the patients.
   D. AChA is duplicated in about 30 % of patients.
   E. MCA has a trifurcation instead of bifurcation in about 20 % of the patients.

✓ The answer is **A**.
- The recurrent artery of Heubner runs parallel to the A1 then parallel to the M1.
- The recurrent artery of Heubner usually arises from A2 segment just distal to Acom in 86–92 % of cases.

❓ 9. Intracranial aneurysms
General relevant anatomy, the FALSE answer is:
   A. The PCA has a fetal origin (arising from the ICA) in 15–22 % of individuals.
   B. The labyrinthine artery arises from AICA in about 85 % of the patients.
   C. Vertebral artery may be hypoplastic and lacking functional significance in 3 % of individuals.
   D. PICA is quite variable and may be absent in about 10 % of individuals.
   E. Artery of Percheron is the name of posterior thalamoperforators when it is bilateral and asymmetric territory.

✓ The answer is **E**.
- The posterior thalamoperforators arise from the P1 segments, with the majority arising from the middle third as individual branches or branching trunks that can be bilateral and symmetric, bilateral and asymmetric, or unilateral with bilateral territory (artery of Percheron).

② 10. Intracranial aneurysms
General cisternal anatomy, the FALSE answer is:
  A. Carotid cistern is containing the ICA and the origin of its branches.
  B. Sylvian cistern is containing the MCA and extends back into the sylvian fissure.
  C. Olfactory cistern is containing the olfactory tract.
  D. Chiasmatic cistern is containing the oculomotor nerve and the pituitary gland.
  E. Lamina terminalis cistern is containing ACA, Acom, and their branches (in the midline).

✔ The answer is D.
  ▬ Chiasmatic cistern is containing the optic nerves, chiasm, and the pituitary stalk (in the midline).
  ▬ Also the interpeduncular cistern is containing Pcom and their branches, the oculomotor nerves, and many components of the basilar artery circulation.

② 11. Intracranial aneurysms
Genetics (autosomal dominant polycystic kidney disease (ADPKD)), the FALSE answer is:
  A. ADPKD accounts for 2–7 % of all intracranial aneurysms.
  B. Intracranial aneurysms are detected in approximately 25 % of patients with ADPKD at autopsy; those are more likely to be male.
  C. Aneurysmal SAH in patients with ADPKD occurs at an earlier age, but the mortality rate is similar.
  D. Renal ultrasonography is a noninvasive and reliable technique and should therefore be considered to rule out ADPKD.
  E. Intracranial aneurysm is detected more likely in male with ADPKD.

✔ The answer is E.
  ▬ Intracranial aneurysm is detected more likely in female with ADPKD.
  ▬ Identifiable heritable connective tissue disorders contribute to a relatively small percentage of intracranial aneurysms.
  ▬ Neurosurgical disorders that have been associated with ADPKD include intracranial aneurysms, cervico-cephalic arterial dissections, intracranial dolichoectasia (abnormally dilated and tortuous artery), intracranial arachnoid cysts, spinal meningeal diverticula/cerebrospinal fluid leaks, and chronic subdural hemorrhages.

- The presence of polycystic liver disease in patients with ADPKD may also increase the development of intracranial aneurysms.
- Patients with ADPLD (autosomal dominant polycystic liver disease) may also be at high risk for the development of intracranial aneurysms.

❷ 12. Intracranial aneurysms
   Genetics, the FALSE answer is:
   A. Intracranial aneurysms may be associated with NF type 2.
   B. An intracranial aneurysm may be the initial manifestation of Ehlers-Danlos syndrome type IV.
   C. Identifying Ehlers-Danlos syndrome type IV in any patient with an intracranial aneurysm is important because vascular fragility can make any invasive procedure a hazardous.
   D. In Marfan's syndrome similar to Ehlers-Danlos syndrome type IV, there is a propensity for proximal intracranial carotid artery involvement.
   E. Coarctation of the aorta, fibromuscular dysplasia, and pheochromocytoma have been associated with intracranial aneurysms.

✓ The answer is **A.**
   - Intracranial aneurysms may be associated with NF type 1 that often coexist with intracranial arterial occlusive disease, thereby increasing the risk associated with the surgical and particularly endovascular treatment of these aneurysms.
   - When Ehlers-Danlos syndrome type IV is suspected, collagen type III analysis should be performed on cultured skin fibroblasts to confirm this diagnosis.

❷ 13. Intracranial aneurysms
   Familial and environmental factors, the FALSE answer is:
   A. Whites are twice more prone to having aneurysms than the black population.
   B. 7–20 % of patients with aneurysmal SAH had first- or second-degree relatives with intracranial aneurysms.
   C. Genetic components may predominate in younger patients.
   D. Environmental components may predominate in the older population.
   E. Cigarette smoking is not a risk factor for intracranial aneurysms.

✓ **The answer is E.**
- Cigarette smoking is the most important modifiable environmental risk factor for intracranial aneurysms. Smokers have a three- to tenfold increased risk for aneurysmal SAH.
- Those who continue to smoke may be at particularly high risk for the de novo development of aneurysms.
- Among first-degree relatives of patients with aneurismal SAH, the risk of a ruptured intracranial aneurysm is approximately four times higher than the risk in the general population.

? **14. Intracranial aneurysms***
Pediatrics, the FALSE answer is:
A. Intracranial aneurysms in childhood account for 1–2 % of intracranial aneurysms.
B. They are different from adults in having a female preponderance.
C. They are different from adults in that ICA being the most common site.
D. They are different from adults in that the MCA bifurcation and the vertebro-basilar system are the second most common site.
E. Posterior circulation aneurysms are more common in children than adults.

✓ **The answer is B.**
- They are different from adults in having a male preponderance.
- There is a predominant male/female ratio approaching 2:1–3:1.
- The reported incidence is higher in females as compared to males, but Lasjaunias reports that the incidence is higher in males up to 2 years of age and, thereafter, the incidence is higher in females.

? **15. Intracranial aneurysms***
Pediatrics, the FALSE answer is:
A. They are different from adults in having a lower incidence of infective, traumatic, and giant aneurysms.
B. The clinical presentation of mass effect or subtle cognitive dysfunction occurs more often than in adults.
C. Presenting symptoms are rather due to the mass effect of the aneurysm than due to aneurysm rupture.
D. Vasospasm associated with hemorrhage is usually well tolerated in the pediatric age group with a relatively low incidence of ischemic deficits.
E. Surgery is usually better tolerated in young children than in adults.

✓ The answer is **A.**
- They are different from adults in having a HIGHER incidence of infective, traumatic, and giant aneurysms.
- Children withstand surgery better than adults due to greater brain functional capacity and better vascular status.
- These patients tend to have lesser incidence of clinical vasospasm and appear to have a better outcome as compared to adults.

16. Intracranial aneurysms
General presentation of unruptured intracranial aneurysm, the FALSE answer is:
   A. Incidental/asymptomatic or minor hemorrhage (sentinel bleed)
   B. CN III palsy or trigeminal neuralgia or visual loss
   C. Seizures (most commonly due to ACA aneurysm)
   D. Headache or migraines (retro-orbital) or endocrine disturbance
   E. Transient ischemic attacks or small infarcts

✓ The answer is **C.**
- Seizures: 5, 10, and 25 % of patients with ruptured anterior, posterior, and MCA aneurysm, respectively, suffered from epilepsy over the course of many years of follow-up.
- CN III palsy: in 9 % of Pcom aneurysms.
- Trigeminal neuralgia: usually in V1 or V2 distribution with intracavernous or supraclinoid aneurysms.
- Visual loss: ophthalmic, Acom, basilar apex aneurysms.
- Endocrine disturbance: due to compression of pituitary stalk or gland by intrasellar or suprasellar aneurysms.
- Transient ischemic attacks or small infarcts: due to distal embolization.

17. Intracranial aneurysms
General presentation, the FALSE answer is:
   A. The most frequent presentation is SAH.
   B. ICH: occurs in 20–40 %.
   C. IVH: occurs in 13–28 %.
   D. SDH: occurs in 2–5 %.
   E. ICH: occurs more common with aneurysms proximal to the circle of Willis.

✓ The answer is **E.**
- ICH: occurs in 20–40 % (more common with aneurysms distal to the circle of Willis, e.g., MCA aneurysms).

? 18. **Intracranial aneurysms**
   Associated IVH, the FALSE answer is:
   A. Acom aneurysm rupture usually causes IVH in the lateral ventricle.
   B. Acom aneurysm rupture usually causes IVH in the third ventricle.
   C. Distal PICA aneurysms rupture usually causes IVH in the third ventricle.
   D. Distal basilar artery aneurysm rupture may cause IVH in the third ventricle.
   E. Carotid terminus aneurysms rupture may cause IVH in the third ventricle.

✓ The answer is **C**.
   - Distal PICA aneurysms usually rupture directly into the **fourth** ventricle through the foramen of Luschka.
   - Acom aneurysm: it has been asserted that IVH occurs from rupture through the lamina terminalis into the anterior third or lateral ventricles; however, this is not always borne out at the time of surgery.
   - Distal basilar artery or carotid terminus aneurysms: may rupture through the floor of the third ventricle (rare).
   - IVH occurs higher in autopsy series and appears to carry a worse prognosis (64 % mortality).
   - The size of the ventricles on admission is the most important prognosticator.

? 19. **Intracranial aneurysms**
   Hemorrhage location in correlation with aneurysm origin, the FALSE answer is:
   A. The frontal horn hemorrhage is related mostly to Pcom aneurysm.
   B. The interhemispheric fissure or gyrus rectus hemorrhage is related mostly to Acom aneurysm.
   C. The sylvian fissure hemorrhage is related mostly to MCA or Pcom aneurysm.
   D. The prepontine or interpeduncular cistern hemorrhage is related mostly to basilar tip or SCA aneurysm.
   E. The prepontine or interpeduncular cistern hemorrhage is sometimes related to perimesencephalic nonaneurysmal SAH.

✓ The answer is **A**.
   - The frontal horn hemorrhage is related mostly to choroidal aneurysm.

? **20.** **Intracranial aneurysms**
General oculomotor palsy in intracranial aneurysm, the
FALSE answer is:
A. Occurs in 9 % of Pcom aneurysm.
B. Occurs less commonly with basilar apex aneurysm.
C. Diplopia and ptosis are the classic findings of third nerve palsy by Pcom aneurysm.
D. Pupil-sparing third nerve palsy is the classic finding of third nerve compression.
E. The development of a third nerve palsy in a patient with an unruptured aneurysm is an emergency result from aneurysmal expansion and impending rupture.

✔ The answer is **D**.
– Non-pupil-sparing third nerve palsy (dilated unreactive pupil) is the classic finding of third nerve compression.

? **21.** **Intracranial aneurysms**
Findings that may suggest impending aneurysm rupture, the FALSE answer is:
A. Progressing cranial nerve palsy
B. Increase in aneurysm size on repeat angiography
C. Partial thrombosis of the aneurysm
D. Beating aneurysm sign
E. Minor hemorrhage

✔ The answer is **C**.
– Partial thrombosis of the aneurysm is not an alarming sign for rupture. IMMINENT ANEURYSM RUPTURE: Findings that may herald impending aneurysm rupture include:
1. Progressing cranial nerve palsy, e.g., development of third nerve palsy with Pcom aneurysm (traditionally regarded as an indication for urgent treatment).
2. Increase in aneurysm size on repeat angiography.
3. Beating aneurysm sign: pulsatile changes in aneurysm size between cuts or slices on imaging (may be seen on angiography, MRA, or CTA).
4. Minor hemorrhage (sentinel bleed) has an average latency of only 11 days between symptom and clinically significant SAH.

? 22. Intracranial aneurysms
Unruptured aneurysms, (5 years cumulative rupture rate), the FALSE answer is:
   A. 2.5 % for 7–12 mm anterior circulation aneurysm
   B. 40 % for 25 mm or more anterior circulation aneurysms
   C. 14 % for 7–12 mm posterior circulation aneurysm
   D. 50 % for 25 mm or more posterior circulation aneurysms
   E. Higher rupture rate in anterior circulation aneurysms

✓ **The answer is E.**
   – Higher rupture rate in posterior circulation aneurysms.
   – The prevalence of UNRUPTURED ANEURYSMS has been found to vary considerably from less than 1 % to as high as 9 %.

? 23. Intracranial aneurysms
Factors associated with rupture, the FALSE answer is:
   A. Aneurysm characteristics associated with rupture include aneurysm size, location, and multiplicity.
   B. Patient characteristics associated with rupture include history of hypertension, previous ischemic cerebrovascular disease, smoking, alcohol, and genetic factors.
   C. Aneurysm growth is unproved relation.
   D. Symptomatic aneurysms is unproved relation.
   E. Men may have an increased likelihood for rupture.

✓ **The answer is E.**
   – Women may have an increased likelihood for rupture.
   – There is an association between the presence of multiple aneurysms and an increased risk for rupture. (The commonest locations for multiple aneurysms are the Pcom and MCA locations.)
   – Increasing age >50 years has been thought to increase the risk for hemorrhage.
   – There is a strong association between cigarette smoking and increased prevalence and risk for rupture.
   – Gender: Women may have an increased likelihood for rupture. In older patients, female rates of subarachnoid hemorrhage are generally 1.5–2.5 times higher than men, and the median age of presentation is later than men. This is largely due to the higher rates of aneurysms in young males.
   – Ethnicity: the high incidences of aneurysmal SAH reported in Japanese or Finnish patients compared to others.
   – Also more in winter and more in daytime.

? 24. **Intracranial aneurysms***
   Incidence of rupture according to the SIZE, the FALSE answer is:
   A. Risk for rupture of <5 mm size unruptured aneurysm is 0.5 % (annual risk).
   B. Risk for rupture of 5–10 mm size unruptured aneurysm is 11.5 % (annual risk).
   C. Risk for rupture of 5–10 mm size unruptured aneurysm is 1.2 % (annual risk).
   D. Risk for rupture of >10 mm size unruptured aneurysm is 1.5 % (annual risk).
   E. Risk for rupture of >15 mm size unruptured aneurysm is 6.1 % (annual risk).

✓ The answer is **B**.
   – Aneurysm size considered to be an important independent variable in the risk for rupture
   – Risks for unruptured aneurysm of different sizes and categorized aneurysms into six not mutually exclusive groups: <5 mm (annual risk 0.5 %), <7 mm (0.4 %), 5–10 mm (1.2 %), >10 mm (1.5 %), >12 mm (3.9 %), and >15 mm (6.1 %)

? 25. **Intracranial aneurysms***
   Factors associated with rupture according to the SITE, the FALSE answer is:
   A. The Pcom is the commonest site of a ruptured aneurysm in surgical series.
   B. A calculated annual risk of rupture for posterior circulation aneurysm is 3.3 %.
   C. A calculated annual risk of rupture for Pcom aneurysm is 2.2 %.
   D. A calculated annual risk of rupture for Acom aneurysm is 1.8 %.
   E. A calculated annual risk of rupture for MCA aneurysm is 1.2 %.

✓ The answer is **A**.
   – The Acom is the commonest site of a ruptured aneurysm in surgical series.
   – Site was an independent variable.
   – The incidence of rupture located at the basilar bifurcation and Pcom locations appears to have a higher risk for rupture than at other sites. In contrast, aneurysms within the cavernous sinus appear to have a lower likelihood of bleeding.
   – Calculated annual risks of rupture by site of aneurysm for the general population are as follows: Acom (1.8 %), ICA (including Pcom 1.3 %), ICA

(excluding Pcom 1.0 %), Pcom (2.2 %), MCA (1.2 %), cavernous ICA (0.1 %), and posterior circulation (3.3 %) (defined as vertebral artery, basilar artery, and PCA). This is supported by the ISUIA (International Study of Unruptured Intracranial Aneurysms) finding that aneurysms of the posterior fossa had higher rupture rates.

26. Intracranial aneurysms
Factors associated with rupture, according to the SHAPE, the FALSE answer is:
A. Neck width, aspect ratio, and bottleneck factor
B. Daughter sacs or blebs or surface irregularity
C. Aneurysm site to parent artery ratio
D. Aneurysm angle to parent artery
E. Aneurysm size to parent artery ratio

The answer is **C.**
- **Neck width**: a 4-mm threshold has been established as defining the neck of saccular aneurysms as small or large.
- **Aspect ratio (height/neck width)**: This parameter is the distance between the neck and the fundus divided by the maximum neck width (sac length, perpendicular to the neck/widest neck width). The larger the ratio value, the longer the aneurysm sac and the greater the likelihood of the aneurysm having ruptured.
- **Neck to sac width ratio (bottleneck factor)**: this parameter (widest sac width/widest neck width) is used to define the likely difficulty of endovascular coil embolization. If the ratio equals 1.0 or less, the aneurysm can be described as sessile in shape and unlikely to retain coils. If greater, the sac is broader than the neck and more favorable for endosaccular packing.
- Volume orifice ratio (aneurysm volume to orifice), i.e., neck area rather than neck width, is a recently described parameter which correlates with whether an aneurysm has ruptured or not.
- Greater than 80 % of aneurysms rupture at the dome.
- Rupture occurs most commonly at the fundus (57–64 %), at a portion of the body (17–33 %), and rarely at the neck region (2–10 %).

27. Intracranial aneurysms
Factors associated with outcome after aneurysm rupture, the FALSE answer is:
A. Hunt and Hess clinical grade on admission is the most important factor.
B. Aneurysm location, time after hemorrhage, gender, age, and hypertension.

C. Rebleeding is not an important risk factor for mortality.
D. The apolipoprotein E genotype (APOE4) would be expressed more frequently in patients with an unfavorable outcome.
E. Smoking is negatively associated with survival after aneurysmal SAH.

✔ The answer is **C**.
  − Rebleeding is strongly correlated with mortality with the rate of rebleeding is highest during the first 24 h then constant at a rate of 1 % per day to 2 % per day over the subsequent 4 weeks.
  − Smoking is positively associated with survival after aneurysmal SAH.
  − The risk of rebleeding from Acom aneurysms is increased by the following factors:
    1. Gender (females)
    2. Aneurysms that point superiorly and have a wide neck
    3. History of coma
    4. Systemic hypertension
    5. Elderly age.
  − The associated risk factors for bleeding from PcomA are different and include:
    1. Age
    2. Larger aneurysms
    3. The presence of clot
    4. Vasospasm

❓ 28. **Intracranial aneurysms**
    General outcome, the FALSE answer is:
    A. About 40 % of patients with ruptured aneurysms die following the SAH, and about 40 % of survivors rebleed in the first year.
    B. The rebleed rate in general is about 3 %, and the death is about 2 % per year.
    C. Severity of the initial SAH is the most important prognostic factor for outcome.
    D. Patients who undergo surgical treatment of paraclinoid aneurysms usually have very poor outcomes.
    E. Surgical outcome for ICA aneurysms is generally good.

✔ The answer is **D**.
  − Patients who undergo surgical treatment of paraclinoid aneurysms usually have good or excellent outcomes.
  − Surgical outcome for ICA aneurysms is generally good, although straightforward cases are no longer treated by surgery, and more complex aneurysms are referred to vascular neurosurgeons.

? **29.** **Intracranial aneurysms**
General management, the FALSE answer is:
A. Now, the management of intracranial aneurysms is based on CTA results, and DSA is requested only in complex aneurysms.
B. Current practice suggests treatment of favorable-grade aneurysms within the first 24–48 h after the SAH.
C. Poor grade patients (WFNS grades IV and V) must get trial of clipping.
D. Routine DSA is done on postoperative day 7–10 to ensure complete obliteration of the aneurysm.
E. If the patient shows clinical evidence of vasospasm, then an angiogram is done.

✓ The answer is **C**.
- Poor grade patients (WFNS grade V and some WFNS grade IV patients) are only treated if they show improvement in SAH grade.
- They are allowed to recover in the intensive care unit with optimization of their electrolytes and antiseizure medications and an external ventricular drain if they have hydrocephalus, and they are only treated if they show improvement in SAH grade. If they are not suitable candidates for endovascular coiling, surgical clipping is performed.

? **30.** **Intracranial aneurysms**
Guidelines for the management of unruptured aneurysm, the FALSE answer is:
A. All asymptomatic intradural aneurysms should be treated.
B. Asymptomatic intracavernous aneurysms are usually better to be observed.
C. Incidental aneurysms with diameters less than 7 mm are usually better to be observed.
D. Endovascular treatment should be considered as a treatment option for incidental aneurysms.
E. Aneurysms located at the Pcom have higher rupture rates and deserve special consideration for treatment.

✓ The answer is **A**.
- All symptomatic intradural aneurysms should be treated.

The other guidelines:
- Aneurysms found in association with a ruptured lesion and those with diameters larger than 7 mm deserve strong consideration for treatment, especially in young patients.

- Aneurysms located at the Pcom and those in the posterior circulation, especially the basilar tip, have higher rupture rates, and therefore deserve special consideration for treatment.

? 31. **Intracranial aneurysms**
   General management (aneurysm clips), the FALSE answer is:
   A. Generally, shorter clips have more closing pressure.
   B. Temporary clips have a closing pressure of 100 mg.
   C. Fenestrated and the right-angled ones are ideal for larger aneurysms with a broad neck, especially at the ICA and basilar tree.
   D. The length of the selected clip should be at least 1.5 times the diameter of the aneurysm neck.
   E. Yasargil clips are cross action clips and popular. Their small shank does not obscure vision.

✓ The answer is **B**.
- Temporary clips differ from permanent clips with their closing pressure not exceeding 25–40 gm.
- As the clip blades flatten the neck, the length of the closed neck will be half of its circumference. Therefore, a 10-mm neck requires at least a 15-mm clip.
- Not infrequently, the clip has to be applied without complete visualization of the hidden vessel and repositioned after decompression of the sac and further dissection.
- Heifetz clips have broader wings with an internal spring action and are preferred for thin, friable walls by some.
- Sugita clips are somewhat similar and come in various angles.
- Malleable clips are used less commonly.

? 32. **Intracranial aneurysms**
   General management (surgery), the FALSE answer is:
   A. Wide splitting of the sylvian fissure should be performed for all aneurysms in the anterior circulation to minimize brain retraction.
   B. Sharp dissection of the neck can result in wide tears that are then difficult to seal.
   C. Either displacement or mobilization of the aneurysm body is usually required to visualize the vessels initially hidden from view.
   D. When dissecting directly on the aneurysm, sharp dissection is better than blunt dissection.
   E. Few Acom aneurysms have necks that are ready to be clipped on initial exposure.

✅ The answer is **B**.
- Blunt dissection of the aneurysm neck can result in wide tears that are then difficult to seal.

❓ 33. **Intracranial aneurysms**
General management; factors that favor surgical clipping, the FALSE answer is:
   A. MCA bifurcation aneurysms
   B. Giant aneurysms or symptoms due to mass effect
   C. Traumatic intracranial aneurysm
   D. Small aneurysm
   E. Wide aneurysm neck

✅ The answer is **C**.
- Giant aneurysms (high recanalization rate with coiling).
- Symptoms due to mass effect: clipping may be better than coiling.
- Small aneurysm (higher incidence of intraprocedural rupture with coiling).
- Other factors favorable for surgical clipping are:
   1. Younger age: lower risk of surgery, and lower lifetime risk of recurrence than with coiling.
   2. Patients with residual filling of the aneurysm after coiling.

❓ 34. **Intracranial aneurysms**
General management; factors that favor coiling, the FALSE answer is:
   A. Posterior circulation aneurysms
   B. Inaccessible ruptured aneurysms
   C. Aneurysm configuration: dome-to-neck ratio of 1:2
   D. Aneurysm configuration: an absolute neck diameter <5 mm
   E. Elderly patients (>75 years.) or patients on clopidogrel or poor clinical grade.

✅ The answer is **C**.
- Aneurysm configuration: dome-to-neck ratio (aka fundus-to-neck ratio 2:1 or more).
- Coiling may be considered in cases where there is a failure of attempted clipping, or with aneurysms that are technically difficult to clip (a category that is very vague and varies widely with the experience of the neurosurgeon).

? 35. **Intracranial aneurysms**
General complications, cranial nerve injury during surgery, the FALSE answer is:
   A. Optic nerve injury during paraclinoid aneurysm surgery.
   B. Oculomotor nerve injury subtemporal approach to the basilar bifurcation.
   C. Fourth, fifth, and sixth nerve injury during transtentorial approach to the basilar trunk.
   D. The combined petrosal approach risks damage to the third nerve.
   E. Lower cranial nerves injury during infratentorial approaches.

✓ The answer is **D**.
  — The combined petrosal approach risks damage to the seventh and eighth nerves.
  — With the subtemporal approach to the basilar bifurcation, about two-thirds of patients sustain third nerve damage. Most recover fully but in some of those, some damage persists.
  — The transtentorial approach to the basilar trunk risks damage to the fourth, fifth, and sixth nerves.
  — Infratentorial approaches may damage the lower cranial nerves, particularly when dissecting and clipping PICA aneurysms. Great care and delicacy are required when retracting these nerves to gain access. Damage can lead to potentially fatal aspiration pneumonia.
  — Prevention of optic nerve injury during paraclinoid aneurysm surgery: While unroofing the optic canal, the dura covering the optic nerve must not be disrupted by the drill. The field is continuously irrigated using saline in order to avoid thermal injury to the optic nerve.

? 36. **Intracranial aneurysms**
General complications, intraoperative rupture, the FALSE answer is:
   A. The two most common causes of intraoperative rupture soon after initiation of the procedure are retraction of brain lobes and dislocation of the parent vessel.
   B. Control is obtained via suction and compression of the bleeding site with cottonoids.
   C. Induced cardiac arrest facilitates quick dissection and application of a pilot clip in case of uncontrolled bleeding.
   D. If the rupture takes place before completing the dissection, permanent clips must be applied to all visualized vessels.
   E. If the rupture takes place before completing the dissection, the aneurysm is prepared for pilot clipping under local flow arrest.

✔ The answer is **D**.
- If the rupture takes place before completing the dissection, temporary clips must be applied to the parent vessels proximally and distally, and the aneurysm is prepared for pilot clipping under local flow arrest.

❓ **37. Intracranial aneurysms**
Pathobiology, features of intracranial vessels may make them more prone to aneurysm formation than extracranial vessels, the FALSE answer is:
A. Fewer elastic fibers in the tunica media
B. Fewer elastic fibers in the tunica adventitia
C. Very thick external elastic lamina
D. Less muscle in the media
E. Thinner adventitia

✔ The answer is **C**.
- No external elastic lamina

❓ **38. Intracranial aneurysms***
Pathobiology, the FALSE answer is:
A. Infundibulum is a funnel-shaped dilation of a vessel's origin with a vessel exiting at the apex of the funnel.
B. Usually dilation of the takeoff of the ophthalmic branch of the ICA.
C. Charcot-Bouchard aneurysms are microaneurysms occurring in the basal ganglia associated with chronic hypertension.
D. Oncotic aneurysms may arise from cerebral embolization of neoplastic cells with cardiac myxomas.
E. Formation of aneurysms following radiation has been reported after treatment of germinoma and medulloblastoma.

✔ The answer is **B**.
- Dilation of the takeoff of a branch of the ICA (usually the Pcom) of 3 mm or less is called an infundibulum. Radiologic and autopsy series suggest an incidence of 6–16 %, which increases with older age. The argument about whether this is a pre-aneurysmal phenomenon or not continues, but it is generally accepted that by itself, an infundibulum does not need to be treated.
- Charcot-Bouchard aneurysms are microaneurysms occurring in small (<300 μm diameter) vessels primarily in the basal ganglia associated with chronic hypertension.

- Oncotic aneurysms may arise from cerebral embolization of neoplastic cells with infiltration of the vessel wall and subsequent aneurysm formation. Thus, the underlying patho-mechanism is quite similar to infectious aneurysms. Subarachnoid or intraparenchymal hemorrhage may result. Neoplastic aneurysms have been reported with cardiac myxoma, choriocarcinoma, and bronchogenic and undifferentiated carcinomas. Treatment consists of resection of the involved segment, if possible, and evacuation of the symptomatic lesion.
- Formation of fusiform aneurysms following radiation and radioactive intrathecal gold therapy has been reported after treatment of germinoma and medulloblastoma. These aneurysms are located in the midline or parasellar region and tend to enlarge and rupture.

? 39. **Intracranial aneurysms**
Neurodiagnostic studies, the FALSE answer is:
A. CT scan is the "gold standard" diagnostic test of aneurysm.
B. MRI may help in the diagnosis of subacute SAH when blood has cleared from the CT scan.
C. MRA has not replaced DSA but is useful to evaluate giant or complex aneurysms and dissections.
D. MRA is useful for partially thrombosed lesions.
E. The four-vessel angiography in multiple projections remains the "gold standard" for diagnosis and treatment planning of aneurysm.

✓ The answer is **A**.
- CT scan is the preferred diagnostic test when a SAH is suspected.
- CTA is useful in large ICH and can eliminate the need for conventional DSA in the rapidly deteriorating patient.
- MRA is useful for partially thrombosed lesions because the internal lumen dimensions visible on DSA may not accurately reflect the aneurysm's true size.

? 40. **Intracranial aneurysms**
Neurodiagnostic studies, the features can be evaluated via the four-vessel angiography, the FALSE answer is:
A. The aneurysm's vessel of origin
B. Aneurysm size, shape, and relationship to parent and adjacent arteries
C. Can assess the location of vasospasm
D. Can suggest mass effect by adjacent vessel displacement
E. The presence of other aneurysms or vascular abnormalities.

✅ The answer is **C**.
- The four-vessel angiography can assess the presence but not the location of vasospasm.

❓ **41. Intracranial aneurysms**
Anesthesia (basic principles and goals), the FALSE answer is:
- A. Anesthesia should be titratable and short acting to permit a prompt controlled wake-up.
- B. Drugs that reduce CBF or increase ICP should be avoided.
- C. Hypotension usually is a must at surgery.
- D. Invasive blood pressure monitoring is necessary in each patient.
- E. Arterial blood gases should be checked during surgery to maintain PaCO2 levels between 30 and 35 mmHg.

✅ The answer is **C**.
- Careful blood pressure control is necessary. Normotension usually is preferred at surgery; however, mean arterial blood pressure should be increased by 10–20 % from the baseline if temporary arterial occlusion is applied. Consequently, invasive blood pressure monitoring is necessary in each patient.
- Arterial blood gases should be checked during surgery to obtain adequate oxygenation and to maintain PaCO2 levels between 30 and 35 mmHg. Lower levels of PaCO2 may decrease CBF, particularly in patients with vasospasm.

❓ **42. Intracranial aneurysms**
Maneuvers for intraoperative brain relaxation, the FALSE answer is:
- A. CSF drainage through an EVD or lumbar drain
- B. Hypoventilation
- C. Head positioning
- D. Osmotherapy
- E. Pharmacologic metabolic suppression

✅ The answer is **B**.
- Hyperventilation.
- The incidence of injury from brain retraction is estimated at **5 %** in intracranial aneurysm procedures.
- CSF drainage through an EVD or lumbar drain. Excessive CSF drainage, however, may be associated with complications.

- Once the dura is opened, CSF also can be drained when the arachnoid is opened during the initial exposure.
- Osmotherapy such as mannitol (0.5–1 g/kg) which may be supplemented with Lasix (10–40 mg). During the initial period (approximately 15 min) of mannitol administration, intravascular volume is increased before urinary output is affected with resultant contracture of the intravascular volume.
- While many neurosurgeons and neuro-anesthesiologists give mannitol upon skin incision, this approach can lead to excessive skin and bone bleeding related to the transient expansion of the intravascular volume.
- Appropriate anesthetic agents.
- Pharmacologic metabolic suppression (e.g., thiopental, propofol).
- Head positioning, including head elevation, and ensuring adequate venous drainage (e.g., chin off chest).
- The role of hypothermia remains controversial.

43. Intracranial aneurysms
Rhoton's anatomic principles directing the surgery, the FALSE answer is:
A. The parent artery should be exposed proximal to the aneurysm.
B. The dissection is carried around the wall of the parent vessel to the origin of the aneurysm.
C. The aneurysmal fundus should be dissected before the neck.
D. The aneurysmal neck should be dissected before the fundus.
E. All perforating arterial branches should be separated from the aneurysmal neck before passing the clip around the aneurysm.

✅ The answer is **C**.

44. Intracranial aneurysms
Rhoton's anatomic principles directing the surgery, the FALSE answer is:
A. The bone flap should be placed as low as possible to minimize brain retraction.
B. A clip with a spring mechanism that allows it to be removed and repositioned should be used.
C. After the clip is applied, the area should always be inspected for kinking or obstruction.
D. If an aneurysm has a broad-based neck that will not easily accept the clip, the neck may be reduced by bipolar coagulation.
E. The use of endoscope to view the neck and perforating branches is crucial in all cases.

✅ The answer is E.

— An endoscopic view of the neck with angled endoscopes may aid by revealing the position of perforating branches not seen in the view provided by the surgical microscope.

1. The parent artery should be exposed proximal to the aneurysm. This allows control of flow to the aneurysm if it ruptures during dissection. Exposure of the ICA above the cavernous sinus will give proximal control for aneurysms arising at the level of the Pcom or AChA. Exposure of the ICA at the level of the ophthalmic and superior hypophyseal arteries is commonly achieved by removing the anterior clinoid process, the adjacent part of the roof of the optic canal, and the posterior part of the orbital roof to gain access to the clinoid segment of the ICA. An operative plan that permits cervical internal carotid occlusion in the neck, either by balloon catheter or by direct exposure, should be considered if anterior clinoid removal and proximal supraclinoid exposure is unlikely to yield adequate proximal control. The supraclinoid carotid or the pre-aneurysmal trunks of the middle cerebral or anterior cerebral arteries should also be exposed initially to obtain proximal control of MCA and ACA aneurysms. The exposure can be directed laterally from the ICA for MCA aneurysms and medially over the optic nerves and chiasm for Acom aneurysms. For basilar apex aneurysms, control of the basilar artery proximal to the aneurysm can be obtained by following the inferior surface of the PCA or the superior surface of the SCA to the basilar artery and then working up the side of the basilar artery to the neck of the aneurysm. An operative plan that includes proximal balloon may also be considered. There are several operative routes, discussed below, under Operative Approaches that increase the length of basilar artery below the apex that can be exposed.

2. If possible, the side of the parent vessel away from or opposite to the site on which the aneurysm arises should be exposed before dissecting the neck of the aneurysm. The dissection can then be carried around the wall of the parent vessel to the origin of the aneurysm.

3. The aneurysmal neck should be dissected before the fundus. The neck is the area that can tolerate the greatest manipulation, has the least tendency to rupture, and is to be clipped. Unfortunately, it is the portion of the aneurysm that is most likely to incorporate the origin of a parent arterial trunk or perforating vessel. Therefore, dissection of the neck and proximal part of the fundus should be performed carefully, with full visualization, to prevent passage of a clip around the parental arterial trunk or significant perforating branches that arise near the neck of the aneurysm. The dissection should not be

started at the dome, because this is the area most likely to rupture before or during surgery.

4. All perforating arterial branches should be separated from the aneurysmal neck before passing the clip around the aneurysm. Before the use of magnification, there was a tendency to keep dissection of aneurysms to a minimum because of the hazard of rupture. The use of magnification has permitted increased accuracy of dissection of the aneurysmal neck and more frequent preservation of the perforating arteries. Thus the risk of occlusion of peri-aneurysmal perforating arterioles that results from placement of a clip on an inadequately exposed aneurysm is greater than the hazard of rupture with microsurgical dissection. Separating perforating arteries from the neck of an aneurysm requires appropriately sized microdissectors. Small spatula dissectors 1- or 2-mm-wide (Rhoton No. 6 or 7) or 40-degree-angle teardrop dissectors are suitable. Separating the perforators, if tightly packed against or adherent to the aneurysm may be facilitated by lowering the blood pressure or by temporary clipping of the parent artery. In other cases, where the middle portion of the body, but not the neck of the aneurysm, can be separated from the perforating arteries, placing a clip around the middle portion will sometimes reduce the width of the aneurysm neck so that the perforators can be separated from the neck before moving the clip to the aneurysm neck. Perforators may also be placed in the open area of a fenestrated clip in some cases where one cannot separate the perforator from the neck. An endoscopic view of the neck with angled endoscopes may aid by revealing the position of perforating branches not seen in the view provided by the surgical microscope.

5. If rupture occurs during microdissection, bleeding should be controlled by applying a small cotton pledget to the bleeding point and concomitantly reducing mean arterial pressure. If this technique does not stop the hemorrhage, temporary occlusion with a clip or occluding balloon can be applied to the proximal blood supply, but only for a brief time.

6. The bone flap should be placed as low as possible to minimize the need for retraction of the brain in reaching the area. Most aneurysms are located on or near the circle of Willis under the central portion of the brain. Cranial-base resection, such as is performed in the orbitozygomatic, anterior petrosectomy, presigmoid, or far-lateral approaches, should be used if it will minimize brain retraction, improve vascular exposure, and broaden the operative angle available for attacking the aneurysm.

7. A clip with a spring mechanism that allows it to be removed, repositioned, and reapplied should be used.
8. After the clip is applied, the area should always be inspected, sometimes with intraoperative angiography, to make certain the clip does not kink or obstruct a major vessel and that no perforating branches are included in it.
9. If an aneurysm has a broad-based neck that will not easily accept the clip, the neck may be reduced by bipolar coagulation. Nearby perforating arteries are protected with a cottonoid sponge during coagulation. The tips of the bipolar coagulation forceps are inserted between adjacent vessels and the neck of the aneurysm and are gently squeezed during coagulation. Short bursts of low current are used, and the tips of the forceps are relaxed and opened between applications of current to prevent them from adhering to the aneurysm and to evaluate the degree of shrinkage.

? 45. Intracranial aneurysms
The main factors influencing craniotomy selection, the FALSE answer is:
A. The aneurysm size
B. The aneurysm location
C. Aneurysm configuration
D. The patient's clinical status
E. The patient's preference

✓ The answer is **E**.
— Surgeon preference is an important factor not the patient preference.
— Of these factors, the **type of aneurysm and its configuration** most influence what craniotomy is used.
— The aneurysm type (e.g., location and size).
— Aneurysm configuration and anatomy of the associated vessels and surrounding osseous and neural structures.

? 46. Intracranial aneurysms
Clear indications for coiling, the FALSE answer is:
A. Anterior circulation aneurysms
B. Posterior circulation aneurysms
C. Multiple aneurysms
D. Paraclinoid aneurysms
E. Aneurysms with severe vasospasm

✔ The answer is **A.**
Other INDICATIONS:
= Patients in extremes of age
= Giant/serpentine, fusiform, dissecting, mycotic, and pseudo-aneurysms
= Blood blister-like aneurysms (Ogawa aneurysms)
= Aneurysms with brain AVM

❓ 47. Intracranial aneurysms
Limitations of endovascular treatment, the FALSE answer is:
A. Tortuosity of neck vessels.
B. Renal failure.
C. Aneurysmal size.
D. Aneurysms with large parenchymal clot may require surgical evacuation and clipping done in the same sitting.
E. Non-availability of modern DSA facility.

✔ The answer is **C.**
= Aneurysmal size is not a real limiting factor.
= Tortuosity of neck vessels (stability of arterial access is the primary step for endovascular treatment).
= Also the high cost of material is one of the limitations.

❓ 48. Intracranial aneurysms
Anterior circulation aneurysm (pterional craniotomy), the FALSE answer is:
A. Most anterior and posterior circulation aneurysms can be approached by pterional craniotomy.
B. Some Acom aneurysms may require minor modifications as orbitozygomatic approach.
C. Carotid-ophthalmic artery aneurysms may require minor modifications as anterior clinoidectomy.
D. For aneurysms that involve the proximal ICA, exposure of the cervical ICA is recommended for proximal control.
E. Acom aneurysm required more degree of position rotation than MCA aneurysms.

✔ The answer is **E.**
= The degree of position rotation depends in part on aneurysm location and anatomy with less rotation for an Acom aneurysm and more rotation for some MCA aneurysms.

? **49. Intracranial aneurysms**
Approaches to MCA aneurysms, the FALSE answer is:
A. Medial transsylvian approach provides early proximal M1 control.
B. Medial transsylvian approach carries high risk of intraoperative rupture when the aneurysm fundus points anteriorly.
C. Lateral transsylvian approach is quicker than a medial transsylvian approach.
D. Lateral transsylvian approach advantage is the aneurysm's neck which can be seen before the dome.
E. Superior temporal gyrus approach is useful for an associated ICH that requires evacuation.

✓ The answer is **D.**
— **Lateral transsylvian:** The disadvantage is the aneurysm's dome which is seen before the neck and M1. The sylvian fissure is dissected from lateral to medial and so this approach is quicker than a medial transsylvian approach; there is less CSF loss because the basal cisterns are not opened, less retraction, and the transsylvian veins may be better preserved. However, the aneurysm's dome is seen before the neck and M1. We prefer this approach when the M1 is very long or for an aneurysm that projects forward to obstruct proximal MCA exposure.
— **Medial transsylvian:** The sylvian fissure is opened from medial to lateral, the ICA followed to its bifurcation, and the MCA trunk defined. This approach provides early proximal M1 control and allows perforators off the M1 to be defined. There are two disadvantages: (1) extensive dissection before the aneurysm is reached, and (2) there is a high risk of intraoperative rupture when the aneurysm fundus points anteriorly and adheres to the sphenoid wing.
— **Superior temporal gyrus:** A 2–3-cm incision that extends posteriorly from just behind the anterior sylvian fissure is made in the superior temporal gyrus parallel to the sylvian fissure. This approach is useful when an ICH requires evacuation or for large aneurysms because it allows circumferential access to the aneurysm and exposure of the aneurysm base and neck while the aneurysm can be retracted.

? **50. Basilar bifurcation (apex) aneurysm**
The FALSE answer is:
A. A right-sided approach is preferable.
B. A left-sided approach is recommended when there is left third nerve palsy.

   C. A left-sided approach is recommended when there is left hemiparesis.

   D. When the bifurcation is located more than 1 cm below the level of the posterior clinoids, the best to use is the subtemporal approach.

   E. Aneurysms located greater than 1 cm above the posterior clinoids cannot be safely exposed through a subtemporal approach.

✔ The answer is **C**.

- For most basilar bifurcation aneurysms, a right-sided approach is preferable.
- A left-sided approach is recommended when there is:
  1. Left third nerve palsy and **right** hemiparesis.
  2. A coexistent left-sided anterior circulation aneurysm and both can be repaired through the same craniotomy.
  3. A left-sided approach may be optimal with an aneurysm oriented to the left.
- The relationship between the basilar artery bifurcation, aneurysm, and the clivus and posterior clinoid process is the major factor that influences surgical approach.
- When the bifurcation is located more than 1 cm below the level of the posterior clinoids, its view often is obscured when using a pterional transsylvian approach, and so these lesions may be better approached using a subtemporal trajectory, modified if necessary with a medial petrosectomy or division of the tentorium to reach down the clivus.
- Lesions at the level of the posterior clinoid and up to 1 cm above the clinoids can be approached using a subtemporal or transsylvian approach. However, the higher the bifurcation is relative to the posterior clinoid, greater temporal lobe retraction is required. Therefore, basilar bifurcation aneurysms located greater than 1 cm above the posterior clinoids cannot be safely exposed through a subtemporal approach and are difficult to reach through a conventional transsylvian or temporopolar approach. Instead, the craniotomy requires modification such as removal of the zygoma or fronto-orbital bone.

❓ 51. **Intracranial aneurysms**

   Temporary artery occlusion during surgery, the FALSE answer is:

   A. Reduce aneurysm fundus pressure

   B. Improve the safety of aneurysm neck dissection

   C. Increase the risk of intraoperative rupture

   D. Help to reduce the increased morbidity and mortality

   E. Allow thrombectomy and aneurysmorrhaphy.

✅ The answer is **C**.

  ▬ Reduce the risk of intraoperative rupture.
  ▬ Temporary occlusion should be kept to a minimum but appropriate use of temporary artery occlusion is an important adjunct during aneurysm surgery.
  ▬ Temporary occlusion of the proximal arteries during surgery will, in most instances, reduce aneurysm fundus pressure. This may improve the safety of aneurysm neck dissection and reduce the risk of intraoperative rupture or help reduce the increased morbidity and mortality that may be associated with intraoperative aneurysm rupture.
  ▬ Temporary occlusion also allows thrombectomy, endoaneurysmectomy, and aneurysmorrhaphy to treat giant and complex aneurysms.

❓ 52. **Intracranial aneurysms**
   Temporary artery occlusion during surgery, the FALSE answer is:
   A. The risk of rupture versus ischemia should be balanced.
   B. Hypotension during temporary occlusion is mandatory.
   C. Perforating vessels patency must be maintained.
   D. Safe occlusion time varies with aneurysm location, patient age, and clinical condition.
   E. Intermittent reperfusion may increase tolerable occlusion time.

✅ The answer is **B**.
There are several basic tenets when temporary occlusion is used:
  ▬ Hypotension during temporary occlusion should be avoided; instead mild hypertension helps collateral flow.
  ▬ Temporary vessel occlusion should be used selectively and the risk of rupture versus ischemia be balanced.
  ▬ Perforating vessels patency must be maintained.
  ▬ Safe occlusion time varies with aneurysm location, patient age, and clinical condition.
  ▬ Intermittent reperfusion may increase tolerable occlusion time.
  ▬ Neuroprotection is recommended. When temporary occlusion is planned or thought likely, intraoperative electrophysiological monitors are necessary.

❓ 53. **Intracranial aneurysms**
   Temporary artery occlusion during surgery, the FALSE answer is:
   A. Pharmacologically induced EEG burst suppression is used.
   B. Mild hypertension is used.

C. Hypothermia is frequently induced.

D. Barbiturates are the most commonly used agent in aneurysm surgery.

E. Total duration of temporary clipping is 45 min.

✅ The answer is **E**.

- Total duration of temporary clipping is 14 min with 0 % radiographic evidence of cerebral infarction (14–21 min 19 %).
- "Neuroprotection" or "cerebral protection" is the use of pharmacologic agents or the manipulation of physiologic parameters to increase resistance to potential damage from temporary focal ischemia. This is best done before occlusion.
- The most common strategy is to decrease the metabolic demand typically through pharmacologically induced EEG burst suppression. Mild hypertension, to increase CBF and promote collateral circulation, or hypothermia frequently is induced during temporary occlusion.
- Barbiturates are the most commonly used agent in aneurysm surgery.

❓ **54. Intracranial aneurysms**
   Intraoperative rupture, the FALSE answer is:
   A. SAH increases the risk of rupture.
   B. Lower initial Hunt and Hess grade increases the risk of rupture.
   C. Attempted aneurysm occlusion before the aneurysm neck is well defined increases the risk of rupture.
   D. Sharp dissection increases the risk of rupture.
   E. Intraoperative rupture can complicate between 5 and 20 % of procedures

✅ The answer is **D**.

- Sharp dissection decreases the risk of uncontrollable rupture.
- Often the consequences of rupture (i.e., size of the hole in the aneurysm) associated with blunt dissection may be worse than sharp dissection.

❓ **55. Carotid ophthalmic artery and paraclinoid ICA aneurysms**
   Operative technique, the FALSE answer is:
   A. Usually cervical ICA exposure done in patients with a clinoidal ICA aneurysm.
   B. Remove the lesser wing of sphenoid.
   C. Remove the ACP (anterior clinoid process).
   D. Remove the PCP (posterior clinoid process).
   E. Remove optic strut (OS).

✅ The answer is **D.**
- Usually cervical ICA exposure done in patients with a clinoidal ICA aneurysm, a complex or giant aneurysm, or aneurysm of the ophthalmic segment.

❓ **56. Paraclinoid aneurysms**
Anatomy, the FALSE answer is:
A. Paraclinoid aneurysms are defined as aneurysms arising from the ICA in close proximity to the ACP.
B. The clinoidal segment is usually devoid of named arterial perforators.
C. Paraclinoid aneurysms are classified according to the segment of origin into clinoidal or ophthalmic segment types.
D. The clinoidal segment is located above and laterals to the ACP.
E. The ophthalmic segment is located above and medial to the ACP.

✅ The answer is **D.**
- The clinoidal segment, the distal portion of the anterior ascending vertical segment of the cavernous carotid artery, is located below and medial to the ACP, above the major venous lumen of the cavernous sinus.
- The ophthalmic segment, the distal portion of the paraclinoid ICA region, lies entirely within the subarachnoid space above and medial to the ACP.

❓ **57. Paraclinoid aneurysms**
Ophthalmic segment, the FALSE answer is:
A. Ophthalmic segment aneurysms include ophthalmic artery aneurysms and superior hypophyseal artery aneurysms.
B. Ophthalmic artery aneurysm rupture rarely causes SAH.
C. Ophthalmic artery aneurysm causes ipsilateral monocular superior nasal quadrantanopia.
D. Ophthalmic artery aneurysm (when giant) causes ipsilateral near-complete loss of vision and contralateral monocular pie in the sky defect.
E. Hypophyseal artery aneurysms include paraclinoid variant and suprasellar variant.

✅ The answer is **B.**
- Ophthalmic artery aneurysms: These lesions typically arise along the posterior bend of the ICA just distal to the ophthalmic artery and dural ring, project dorsally or dorsomedially, and elevate the lateral edge of the optic nerve against the falciform ligament. The pressure from the falciform

ligament against the superior surface of the nerve results in an inferior nasal field defect.
- Ophthalmic artery aneurysm presentation:
  1. 45 % present as SAH.
  2. 45 % present as visual field defect:
     A. As the aneurysm enlarges, it impinges on the lateral portion of the optic nerve which causes inferior temporal fiber compression that causes ipsilateral monocular superior nasal quadrantanopia.
     B. Continued enlargement causes upward displacement of the nerve against the falciform ligament which causes superior temporal fiber compression that causes monocular inferior nasal quadrantanopia.
     C. In addition to near-complete loss of vision in the involved eye, compression of the optic nerve near the chiasm may produce a superior temporal quadrant defect in the contralateral eye (junctional scotoma aka "pie in the sky" defect) from injury to the anterior knee of Willebrand (nasal retinal fibers that course anteriorly for a short distance after they decussate in the contralateral optic nerve).
  3. 10 % present as both
- Superior hypophyseal artery aneurysms: There are two main variants:
  1. The parasellar variant projects inferiorly toward the sella into the carotid cave, whereas the suprasellar variant projects superiorly into the suprasellar space. Parasellar superior hypophyseal artery aneurysms (also been called carotid cave aneurysms) are usually asymptomatic.
  2. Suprasellar or large lesions have a much higher tendency to rupture. When large or giant, these aneurysms tend to elevate the optic chiasm and produce visual changes and relationships to the visual system similar to those seen with pituitary tumors.

❷ 58. Paraclinoid aneurysms
Ophthalmic and clinoidal segments, the FALSE answer is:
   A. Aneurysms from both of these carotid segments are much more common in males.
   B. These segments have a propensity for aneurysm multiplicity.
   C. Most paraclinoid aneurysms have a lower rupture risk compared with those at other intracranial subarachnoid sites.
   D. Most large (≥1 cm) clinoidal segment aneurysms carry an increased risk for intracranial hemorrhage.
   E. Small clinoidal segment aneurysms may be cured with endovascular coiling only.

✅ The answer is **A**.

- Aneurysms from both of these carotid segments are much more common in women, with ratios as high as 9:1 female-to-male predominance.
- Most present during the fifth and sixth decades of life, usually as either incidental lesions or with mass effect.
- These segments have a propensity for aneurysm multiplicity; up to half of ophthalmic segment aneurysm patient harbor at least one additional intracranial aneurysm.
- With the exception of the dorsal variant, which often represents an unstable dissection, most paraclinoid aneurysms have a lower rupture risk compared with those at other intracranial subarachnoid sites.
- Small asymptomatic aneurysms (<1 cm) are intradural below the subarachnoid space and are therefore generally treated conservatively.
- Small symptomatic lesions and lesions whose protective ACP roof has been removed for treatment of another aneurysm in the region should be treated.
- Most large (≥1 cm) clinoidal segment aneurysms have extended through the overlying dural coverings into the subarachnoid space and carry an increased risk for intracranial hemorrhage, and stronger consideration for intervention is therefore given to such lesions even if asymptomatic.
- Large or giant clinoidal segment lesions often require coiling combined with stenting to achieve satisfactory aneurysm obliteration. Direct surgical obliteration is also a reasonable option but requires broad removal of the ACP and optic strut and opening of the dural ring to gain satisfactory exposure for accurate clip placement. Lesions presenting with epistaxis should be obliterated urgently.
- Many small unruptured ophthalmic segment lesions appear to have very low risk for rupture, particularly the parasellar superior hypophyseal artery variant, and conservative or endovascular treatment is often preferable to surgery, particularly in older patients with higher surgical risks. When surgery is done, early sectioning of the falciform ligament is helpful to prevent iatrogenic optic nerve injury.

❓ 59. **Paraclinoid aneurysms**
   Ophthalmic segment, operative technique, the FALSE answer is:
   A. Anterior clinoidectomy has great value in the surgical exposure for most paraclinoid aneurysms.
   B. The extradural anterior clinoidectomy is preferable.

C. The risk of damaging the adjacent perforating branches is less in clipping an ophthalmic aneurysm than at other sites on the ICA.
D. The origin of the ophthalmic artery is difficult to expose because of its short intradural length and its location under the optic nerve.
E. Perforator injury during superior hypophyseal artery aneurysm clipping can lead to visual loss.

✓ The answer is **B**.

- The intradural anterior clinoidectomy is preferable in most instances because it allows the surgeon to see the optic nerve and aneurysm during the entire dissection.
- The risk of damaging the adjacent perforating branches is less in clipping an ophthalmic aneurysm than at other sites on the ICA because ophthalmic aneurysms typically point upward, away from these perforating branches.
- Perforator injury during superior hypophyseal artery aneurysm clipping can lead to visual loss, so most superior hypophyseal artery aneurysms are best clipped using fenestrated clips.

❓ 60. **Paraclinoid aneurysms**
Surgery, the FALSE answer is:
A. The AChA is seen before the Pcom, although the AChA arises after to the Pcom.
B. The AChA is seen before because the supraclinoidal ICA passes in more lateral direction.
C. The AChA is seen before because it arises further laterally on the posterior wall of the carotid than the Pcom.
D. AChA arises proximal to the Pcom.
E. The AChA pursues a more lateral course than the Pcom.

✓ The answer is **D**.

- In exposing the carotid artery beyond the origin of the ophthalmic artery, the surgeon often sees the AChA before the Pcom, although the AChA arises distal to the Pcom. This occurs because of three sets of anatomic circumstances.
  1. First, the supraclinoid segment of the ICA passes upward in a posterolateral direction, placing the origin of the more distally arising branch, the AChA, and further lateral to the midline than the origin of the Pcom, which arises more proximally.

2. Second, the AChA arises further laterally on the posterior wall of the carotid than the Pcom.

3. Third, the AChA pursues a more lateral course than the Pcom; the former passes laterally below the optic tract, around the cerebral peduncle, and into the temporal horn, whereas the latter is directed in a posteromedial direction above and medial to the oculomotor nerve toward the interpeduncular fossa. Care should be taken to preserve both the Pcom and the AChA at the time of obliteration of ICA aneurysms. Occlusion of either of these arteries may cause a hemiplegia, homonymous hemianopia, and reduced levels of consciousness.

❓ 61. Paraclinoid aneurysms
Post-op visual complication, the FALSE answer is:
A. Visual symptoms are worsened in 0–8 % after surgical clipping.
B. Visual symptoms improved in 50–74 % after surgical clipping.
C. The cause of worsened vision is vascular in most of the cases.
D. Mechanical injury may occur from manipulation of the optic nerve against the falciform ligament.
E. Thermal injury can occur during drilling of the anterior clinoid process.

✅ The answer is **C**.
- The cause of worsened vision can be mechanical, thermal, or rarely vascular (perforator injury).
- Visual symptoms improved in 50–74 %, remained stable in 26–42 %, and are worsened in 0–8 % after surgical clipping.

❓ 62. Paraclinoid aneurysms*
Carotid cave aneurysms, the FALSE answer is:
A. The carotid cave is a short downward pouching, extends a variable distance below the level of the upper dural ring of the ICA.
B. The carotid cave is most prominent on the posterolateral side of the ICA.
C. Carotid cave aneurysms are those located above the upper ring, but extending into the cave adjacent the upper ring.
D. If the aneurysm arises in the carotid cave, the fundus will extend upward out of the carotid cave on the anteromedial aspect of the ICA.
E. The cave seems to become less prominent as the arteries elongate with advancing age.

✅ The answer is **B**.

- The carotid cave is most prominent on the anteromedial side of the ICA.
- The upper ring forms a tight collar around the artery, but inspection under the operating microscope reveals that there is often a narrow depression in the dura at the site at which the ring hugs the anteromedial aspect of the artery, called the carotid cave.
- Carotid cave aneurysms are distinct from clinoid segment aneurysms, which arise from the clinoid segment of the ICA located between the upper and lower dural ring.
- Aneurysms that arise from the clinoid segment of the ICA have been referred to as clinoid segment aneurysms, and those located above the upper ring, but extending into the cave adjacent the upper ring, are referred to as carotid cave aneurysms.

❓ 63. **POSTERIOR COMMUNICATING (Pcom) aneurysms**
Anatomy, the FALSE answer is:
   A. The communicating segment of the ICA begins just below the Pcom artery and ends at the bifurcation.
   B. Two major arterial branches (the Pcom artery and the AChA) arise from communicating segment.
   C. The Pcom arises from the posteromedial surface of the ICA.
   D. The Pcom courses below and lateral to the oculomotor nerve.
   E. The Pcom joins the PCA at the junction of the P1 and P2 segments.

✅ The answer is **D**.

- The Pcom courses medially and inferiorly, through the membrane of Liliequist, above and medial to the oculomotor nerve.

❓ 64. **Pcom aneurysms**
Anatomy, the FALSE answer is:
   A. Multiple perforators arise from the Pcom and are named the anterior thalamic perforators.
   B. These perforators can be stuck to the aneurysm.
   C. These perforators should not be clipped with the aneurysm.
   D. In about 20 % of patients, there is fetal origin of PCA.
   E. In case of fetal origin, the Pcom can be sacrificed.

✅ The answer is **E**.

- In case of fetal origin, the Pcom cannot be sacrificed, and the aneurysm must be clipped in a way to guarantee patency of the parent vessel.
- In about 20 % of patients, the P1 segment of the PCA is hypoplastic, and the PCA arises directly from the Pcom. This is called fetal origin of PCA.

? 65. Pcom aneurysms
Anatomy, the FALSE answer is:
A. The typical Pcom aneurysm arises just distal to the origin of the artery from the wall of the ICA and hence is classified as an ICA aneurysm.
B. The Pcom aneurysm projects posteriorly, laterally, and slightly inferiorly and may pinch the oculomotor nerve as it enters the dural fold of cavernous sinus.
C. The third nerve palsy usually occurs with an acutely expanded Pcom aneurysm.
D. RAH is the most important branch associated with Pcom aneurysms.
E. AChA is lying adjacent to the distal neck.

✓ The answer is **D**.
- AChA is the most important branch associated with Pcom aneurysms, lying adjacent to the distal neck.
- The general rule is to preserve the Pcom and the fetal Pcom; however, if the preoperative angiogram ensures the absence of ipsilateral fetal origin of the PCA and confirms filling of the artery from the posterior circulation, the origin of the Pcom may be included in the clip (if there is no other alternative). This is followed by a second clip applied between the aneurysm and the first thalamoperforators.

? 66. Pcom aneurysms
Presentation, the FALSE answer is:
A. More common in females.
B. They usually cause symptoms when larger than 10 mm in patients with SAH.
C. They usually cause IVH into the temporal horn.
D. They could expand and compress the third cranial nerve, causing painful non-pupil-sparing oculomotor nerve palsy.
E. The likelihood of rupture for Pcom is higher than that associated with posterior circulation aneurysms.

✓ The answer is **E**.
- The International Study of Unruptured Intracranial Aneurysms (ISUIA) has shown a likelihood of rupture for this location, similar to that associated with posterior circulation aneurysms.
- Third nerve palsy following SAH or rapid expansion of a Pcom aneurysm usually resolves completely after 3 months in up to 90 % of patients and resolves partially in the remaining 10 %.

? 67. Pcom aneurysms
Surgical principles, the FALSE answer is:
A. Avoid temporal lobe retraction because this may avulse an aneurysm stuck to the temporal lobe.
B. The clip blades usually risk both AChA and trochlear nerve.
C. Must identify the AChA.
D. The ICA should not be retracted medially away from the aneurysm because this may rupture an adherent dome.
E. Ensure that the clip blades are not too long to prevent oculomotor nerve injury.

✔ The answer is **B**.
− The clip blades usually risk both AChA and oculomotor nerve.

? 68. ANTERIOR CHOROIDAL ARTERY (AChA) aneurysms
Anatomy, the FALSE answer is:
A. According to the Bouthillier classification of ICA segments, aneurysms of the AChA arise from the C7 segment, which is also called the posterior communicating segment.
B. According to commonly used classification, AChA arises from choroidal segment, which begins at the takeoff of the AChA and ends at the carotid bifurcation.
C. AChA arises proximal and lateral to the Pcom.
D. AChA following course of the optic tract.
E. The main trunk of AChA continues posteriorly, inferior to the optic tract, to enter the choroid fissure.

✔ The answer is **C**.
− AChA arises distal and lateral to the Pcom.
− AChA has a characteristic course, swinging initially laterally and then posteriorly, following the optic tract and supplying a branch to the mesial temporal structures.
− The size of this artery is variable, and duplication occurs in as many as 30 % of normal autopsy specimens.

? 69. AChA aneurysms
Presentation, the FALSE answer is:
A. AChA aneurysms may be difficult to differentiate radiologically from Pcom aneurysm.
B. IVH usually involves the frontal horn.

   C. Because of high location of the AChA above the tentorium, cranial nerve deficits are unlikely.

   D. Usually, there is a risk for endovascular coiling of the AChA.

   E. These aneurysms are often referred for surgical treatment.

✅ The answer is **B**.
- IVH usually involves the temporal horn.

❓ **70. AChA aneurysms**
Operative technique, the FALSE answer is:
   A. Excessive temporal lobe retraction is avoided because it may rip the dome.
   B. In 70 % of the cases, the AChA arises as a single trunk.
   C. The key to this operation is to preserve the AChA.
   D. Occlusion of AChA may lead to contralateral hemiparesis only.
   E. There is no reliable technique to confirm the patency of the AChA after clipping.

✅ The answer is **D**.
- Occlusion of AChA artery leads to classic triad of contralateral hemiparesis, hemianopia, and hemisensory deficit.
- Excessive temporal lobe retraction is avoided because it may rip the dome of the AChA aneurysm, which frequently adheres to the mesial temporal lobe.
- Unfortunately, there is no reliable technique to confirm the patency of the AChA except for the direct visualization and inspection of flow inside the artery.

❓ **71. ICA bifurcation aneurysms**
Anatomy and presentation, the FALSE answer is:
   A. The bifurcation of the ICA into an ACA and MCA takes place beneath the basal forebrain and the anterior perforated substance.
   B. The aneurysm usually points anterosuperiorly.
   C. In most cases, the lenticulostriate perforators of the ICA are displaced posteriorly and may be adherent to the aneurysm.
   D. Most commonly present with SAH, but they may present with ICH into the basal ganglia, simulating hypertensive hemorrhage.
   E. Most are favorable for coiling procedure.

✅ The answer is **E**.
- Most have a broad base, making an unassisted coiling procedure less favorable.

72. ICA bifurcation aneurysms
   The FALSE answer is:
   A. The ICA bifurcation aneurysms constitute 5 % of all intracranial aneurysms with a male predominance.
   B. The ICA bifurcation is the commonest site in children, and they have a worse outcome than their adult counterparts.
   C. The dome of the aneurysm, which is usually buried into the substance of the basal forebrain, should not be disturbed.
   D. A small frontal corticotomy may be performed to facilitate visualization of the lenticulostriate and the recurrent artery of Heubner.
   E. Usually, a straight clip or laterally angled straight clip is applied perpendicular to the direction of ACA and MCA.

The answer is **B**.
   — The ICA bifurcation is the commonest site in children, and they have a **better outcome** than their adult counterparts.
   — Multiple aneurysms are seen in 43 % of patients and the most frequent site of another aneurysm is on the MCA.
   — Bilateral ICA bifurcation aneurysms occur in 6 %.

73. Blister aneurysms of ICA*
   The FALSE answer is:
   A. The blood blister-like aneurysms are thin-walled, broad-based aneurysms that lack an identifiable neck.
   B. They are fragile and can rupture during microsurgery.
   C. The diagnosis of these rare aneurysms is crucial before surgery because the strategy for treatment is different from that of saccular aneurysms.
   D. They are mostly asymptomatic and do not necessitate treatment.
   E. 3D CTA can easily detect these aneurysms.

The answer is **D**.
   — They are mostly present with SAH and necessitate treatment.
   — They are fragile and can rupture during microsurgery, causing postoperative rebleeding more frequently than saccular aneurysms.

74. Blister aneurysms of ICA*
   The FALSE answer is:
   A. Endovascular embolization is not recommended.
   B. They are usually large based and the very loose fibrinous tissue at the dome.

C. Application of an encircling clip is limited, because of possible sacrifice of the perforating vessel.
D. If clipping is not successful, carotid sacrifice by trapping with or without revascularization should be done.
E. The most successful option is wrapping materials alone around the aneurysms.

✓ The answer is **E**.
- The success rate after wrapping alone is low because of the fragility and likelihood of further growth.

❓ 75. Anterior cerebral and anterior communicating artery (ACA and Acom) aneurysms
Anatomy, the FALSE answer is:
A. The most important perforator from the ACA segment is the RAH.
B. The RAH arises from the A2 segment in 78 % of cases.
C. The RAH courses anterior or superior to the A1 segment.
D. The RAH will be encountered after the A1 segment on initial retraction of the frontal lobe during surgery in most cases.
E. The length of the RAH is on average twice that of the A1 segment. Its length therefore increases its exposure to injury during surgery.

✓ The answer is **D**.
- The RAH will be encountered before the A1 segment on initial retraction of the frontal lobe during surgery in most cases.
- The most important perforator from the proximal A2 segment is the medial striate artery, better known as the recurrent artery of Heubner (RAH).

❓ 76. ACA and Acom aneurysms
Anatomy, the recurrent artery of Heubner, the FALSE answer is:
A. It is unique among arteries in that it doubles back on its parent vessel.
B. The RAH supplies the anterior limb of the internal capsule.
C. Injury to RAH typically results in a moderate paresis of the contralateral upper extremity and mild paresis of the contralateral face.
D. Injury to RAH never causing aphasia.
E. It also causes dysfunction of the tongue and palate.

✅ The answer is **D**.
- If the dominant hemisphere is involved, an expressive aphasia may be evident.
- It also causes dysfunction of the tongue and palate, which can only be documented during a careful swallowing evaluation.
- In most patients, these deficits tend to resolve completely in a matter of months.
- It is unique among arteries in that it doubles back on its parent vessel, passing above the carotid bifurcation, before entering the anterior perforated substance.
- The RAH supplies anterior striatum (caudate nucleus and putamen), a portion of the outer segment of globus pallidus, and anterior limb of internal capsule.

❓ 77. Acom aneurysms
The FALSE answer is:
A. The Acom aneurysm forms the largest percentage of ruptured aneurysms.
B. Acom and ACA aneurysms are more common in males.
C. These aneurysms are seen in the middle aged.
D. These aneurysms are seen with a peak in the late forties.
E. The "Acom aneurysm syndrome" includes memory disturbance, confabulation, paraparesis, and personality changes.

✅ The answer is **B**.
- Acom and ACA aneurysms are more common in females.

❓ 78. Acom aneurysms
RADIOLOGY, the FALSE answer is:
A. CT alone can lead to diagnosis which is unique for this aneurysm.
B. Characteristic CT scan findings are either SAH mainly in the interhemispheric fissure or a thick clot in the interhemispheric fissure or ICH in the gyrus rectus.
C. IVH is very rare.
D. Acom aneurysm has the highest false-negative rate of angiography of any intracranial aneurysm.
E. Acute hydrocephalus was present in 25 % of patients.

✅ The answer is **C**.
- IVH is seen in up to 79 % of cases, with the blood entering the ventricles from the ICH in about one third of these.
- SAH in these aneurysms results in blood in the anterior interhemispheric fissure in essentially all cases and is associated with ICH in 63 % of cases.
- Acom aneurysm has the highest false-negative rate of angiography of any intracranial aneurysm (due to the balanced flow into the Acom from the paired A1 segments, which may prevent filling of the aneurysm by the dye).

❓ **79. Acom aneurysms**
The FALSE answer is:
A. Acom aneurysm complex exhibits considerable anatomic variation like "dominance" of one A1 segment.
B. The aneurysm usually points in the direction of flow, so may be approached best from the dominant A1.
C. When there is large ICH, the approach is from the side of the ICH to remove the clot.
D. The initial dissection occurs on the anterior surface of the A1 segment taking care to avoid the AChA.
E. Gyrus rectus resection is being helpful especially in superiorly oriented aneurysms to visualize both A2.

✅ The answer is **D**.
- The initial dissection then occurs on the anterior surface of the A1 segment taking care to avoid the recurrent artery of Heubner.
- Acom aneurysm complex exhibits considerable anatomic variation. In particular, "dominance" of one A1 segment (i.e., a large-caliber A1 vessel supplies the aneurysm, whereas the opposite A1 is hypoplastic) is seen. The aneurysm usually points in the direction of flow (i.e., away from the dominant A1 and toward the opposite hemisphere) and so may be approached best from the dominant A1. When there is ICH, particularly one that causes mass effect in the basal-frontal region, the approach is from the side of ICH to remove clot.
- In the presence of an Acom aneurysm, the paired A1 segments are of unequal diameter in as many as 85 % of cases.
- The Acom is rarely oriented in a strictly transverse plane and only in 18 % of cases do ACAs enter the interhemispheric fissure side by side. Thus the Acom is usually oriented in an oblique or sagittal plane.
- Most Acom aneurysms (71.2 %) project into the interhemispheric fissure and only 16 % of all Acom aneurysms has complex, multilobulated projections.

? 80. Acom aneurysms
   The FALSE answer is:
   A. Superior projecting aneurysm obscures the contralateral A1/A2 junction.
   B. Anterior projecting aneurysm obscures the contralateral optic nerve.
   C. Posterior projecting aneurysm obscures the takeoff of the contralateral A2.
   D. Inferior projecting aneurysm obscures the hypothalamic perforating arteries.
   E. Posterior projecting aneurysm obscures the contralateral optic nerve.

✓ The answer is **E.**
To understand dissection, Acom aneurysms may be classified into one of four projections based on their orientation in true anatomic space:
- **Superior:** Aneurysms project into the interhemispheric fissure, and the fundus often obscures the contralateral A1/A2 junction. Fundus depression during microdissection will help identify the contralateral A1 segment.
- **Anterior:** these lesions fill the space between the two optic nerves and so may obscure the contralateral optic nerve.
- **Posterior:** Aneurysms project both above and below the plane formed by the A2 segments and often obscure the takeoff of the contralateral A2. Fenestrated clips are useful to occlude this type of Acom aneurysm.
- **Inferior:** These aneurysms are "under" the Acom in the region of the hypothalamic perforating arteries that arise from the Acom. The Acom complex vessels generally can be defined before clip application; however, these lesions may be dangerous because there is an intimate association with the perforating vessels and a difficult clip angle.

? 81. Acom aneurysms
   The FALSE answer is:
   A. Microsurgical clip application is the preferred option in the treatment of Acom with anteriorly directed fundi.
   B. Endovascular packing is usually selected for Acom with posteriorly directed fundi.
   C. Acom are surgically challenging lesions because of their unilateral retrograde arterial supply.
   D. Acom are surgically challenging lesions because of their intimate relationship to 11 critical arteries and perforators.
   E. Acom are surgically challenging lesions because of their deep and midline location.

✅ The answer is **C**.
- ▬ Acom are surgically challenging lesions because of their bilateral antegrade arterial supply.
- ▬ Their intimate relationship to **11 critical arteries and their perforators**:
- ▬ Two A1 segments
- ▬ Two A2 segments
- ▬ Two medial striate arteries of Heubner
- ▬ Two orbitofrontal arteries
- ▬ Two frontopolar arteries
- ▬ The Acom
- ▬ There is no other aneurysm intimately associated with as many vessels. Meticulous preservation of all these vessels is the supreme challenge of clipping Acom aneurysms.
- ▬ The Acom typically have only one parent artery (unlike most other intracranial aneurysms).
- ▬ Although Acom aneurysms are midline structures, they are nevertheless best approached through a lateral craniotomy, and both A1 segments have to be exposed early in the dissection to obtain proximal control.

❓ 82. **Acom aneurysms**
Operative technique, the FALSE answer is:
A. Opening of three arachnoid cisterns (carotid, chiasmatic, and lamina terminalis) lead to the Acom.
B. Resection of the gyrus rectus is essential for adequate exposure of most Acom.
C. Opening of the lamina terminalis is better to be done before the aneurysm clipping in all cases.
D. Aneurysms up to 1 cm from the Acom may be approached through a standard pterional craniotomy with partial gyrus rectus resection.
E. Anterior-pointing aneurysms have the most favorable surgical anatomy.

✅ The answer is **C**.
- ▬ Opening of the lamina terminalis increases brain relaxation intraoperatively and reduces the incidence of post-SAH chronic hydrocephalus, but may have to be delayed after the aneurysm is clipped because an inferior-pointing aneurysm may obstruct access to the lamina terminalis, or the dome of a posterior-pointing aneurysm may be prematurely decompressed with this maneuver.

- Anterior-pointing aneurysms have the most favorable anatomy in this respect because the critical infundibular and hypothalamic perforators course in a direction opposite the aneurysm.
- Aneurysms >1 cm distal to the Acom up to the genu of the corpus callosum, including those of the pericallosal-callosomarginal bifurcation, may be approached surgically by a basal frontal interhemispheric approach via a frontal craniotomy.

83. Acom aneurysms
Complications, the FALSE answer is:
A. The Acom aneurysm is frequently complicated by electrolyte disturbance.
B. The most common electrolyte abnormality in these patients is hypernatremia.
C. The hyponatremia is commonly due to cerebral salt wasting syndrome rather than SIADH.
D. The Acom aneurysm is frequently complicated by cognitive dysfunction.
E. Cognitive dysfunction is usually the result of a focal lesion in the basal forebrain.

The answer is **B**.
- The most common electrolyte abnormality in these patients is hyponatremia.

84. Acom aneurysms
Selection criteria for endovascular treatment, the FALSE answer is:
A. An absent A1 segment is a reason for concern but not an absolute contraindication to endovascular therapy.
B. Anatomic features associated with complete embolization included small aneurysm size (<10 mm), small neck size (<4 mm), and anterior dome projection.
C. Factors associated with aneurysm recanalization included large size, posterior dome orientation, and incomplete embolization.
D. Endovascular coiling should be selected as the treatment choice for anteriorly directed domes.
E. Higher rates of surgical complication are found with posteriorly projecting domes.

✅ The answer is **D**.

— Endovascular coiling should be selected as the treatment choice for posteriorly directed domes.

— The only morphologic risk factor associated with microsurgical treatment was aneurysm dome orientation, with higher rates of surgical complication found with posteriorly projecting domes.

❓ 85. **Acom aneurysms**
   OUTCOME, the FALSE answer is:
   A. Acom have the best surgical outcomes among all anterior circulation aneurysms.
   B. The clinical grade of the patient as measured by the Hunt and Hess or WFNS scale is the primary factor that determines the final outcome.
   C. Most of the posterosuperior pointing aneurysms presented in poorer grades.
   D. Outcome of the posterosuperior pointing aneurysms is usually unsatisfactory.
   E. The most important predictor of outcome was a postoperative stroke.

✅ The answer is **A**.

— Acom have worst surgical outcomes among all anterior circulation aneurysms.

— The majority of patients surgically treated for SAH reported psychosocial and neurobehavioral changes that were disabling for them and burdensome to their family.

— In comparison most of the anteroinferiorly pointing aneurysms presented in a better grade and the results were satisfactory.

— About 75 % of poor outcomes were due to a major ischemic stroke.

❓ 86. **Distal anterior cerebral artery aneurysms (DACA)**
   The FALSE answer is:
   A. DACA arise on the ACA or its branches distal to the Acom.
   B. They are uncommon pathologic entity.
   C. Typically, these aneurysms are giant and narrow neck in conformation.
   D. The callosomarginal artery (CMA) is the most common site of DACA.
   E. CMA originates most frequently from the A3 segment.

✅ The answer is **C**.

- ▬ Typically, these aneurysms are **small and broad** based in conformation.
- ▬ The callosomarginal artery originates most frequently (2/3 of cases) from the A3 segment, an average of 43 mm from the Acom junction.
- ▬ The frontopolar artery is the second most common site of DACA. And less commonly at the site of origin of orbitofrontal branch of the ACA.

❓ 87. **DACA**
The FALSE answer is:
A. Giant aneurysms in this region are exceedingly rare.
B. DACA are associated with additional intracerebral aneurysms at rates as high as 20–25 %.
C. DACA are very rarely spontaneous saccular aneurysm.
D. DACA can be mycotic aneurysms.
E. DACA can be traumatic or tumorous aneurysms.

✅ The answer is **C**.

- ▬ DACA most commonly are spontaneous saccular aneurysm.
- ▬ In fact, in contrast to typical aneurysms in other anatomic locations, many of the ruptured DACA are found to be less than 5 mm in diameter, and giant aneurysms in this region are exceedingly rare.
- ▬ An additional critical feature of DACA is their common association with additional intracerebral aneurysms, occurring at rates as high as 20–25 % in large series. These other aneurysms are usually found either on the MCA or at the bifurcations of the ICA.

❓ 88. **DACA**
The FALSE answer is:
A. Traumatic aneurysms are thought to result from shearing forces exerted on the distal pericallosal artery at the lower margin of falx cerebri.
B. Aneurysms that arise from tumor emboli are most commonly in atrial myxomas.
C. These aneurysms are often requiring microsurgical clipping of the neck.
D. These aneurysms are often requiring trapping with vessel sacrifice.
E. The most commonly observed variants in distal ACA anatomy is azygous ACA.

✅ The answer is **C**.
- These aneurysms may not be amenable to classic microsurgical clipping of the neck and often require trapping with vessel sacrifice.
- The observed variants in distal ACA anatomy include azygous ACA (type I variation), up to 10 % of DACA are associated with an azygous ACA, in which the distal segments of both anterior cerebral arteries are represented by a single common vessel.
- The presence of azygous ACA has significant implications, both in considering the surgical approach and in clinical outcome, because damage to the single trunk may result in bihemispheric deficits.

❓ 89. **DACA**
   CLINICAL PRESENTATION, the FALSE answer is:
   A. The average age at presentation of patients with DACA is about 50 years.
   B. DACA appears to have a slight female preponderance.
   C. Patients with a ruptured DACA present with classic findings of SAH.
   D. ICH is very rare complication of ruptured DACA.
   E. All patients with ruptured DACA should search for additional aneurysms.

✅ The answer is **D**.
- ICH is a common complication of ruptured DACA and may be found in as many as 50 % of cases.
- SAH (which is often prominent in the interhemispheric fissure across the top of the corpus callosum).
- All patients with suspected ruptured DACA should undergo four-vessel angiography in an attempt to identify the ruptured aneurysm as well as to uncover additional aneurysms.

❓ 90. **DACA**
   MANAGEMENT, the FALSE answer is:
   A. DACA are often treated microsurgically because of their peripheral location, small size.
   B. DACA are often treated microsurgically because of their unfavorable neck-to-parent artery ratio, tendency to "blow out" the bifurcation at which they occur.
   C. The amount of brain retraction needed to clip these lesions is more than other aneurysms.

D. Factors that favor endovascular treatment include extreme age, significant medical comorbidities, poor neurological condition, and irreversible coagulopathy.

E. Proximal arterial control is always achieved later with approach to DACA than with traditional skull base approaches.

✅ The answer is **C**.

— The amount of brain retraction and muscle dissection needed to clip these lesions is comparatively minimal relative to other aneurysms.

❓ **91. Middle cerebral artery (MCA) aneurysms**
The FALSE answer is:

A. The MCA is the third most common location of all intracranial aneurysms.

B. The MCA usually arise at the M1/M2 junction.

C. MCA aneurysms are unique because they may grow to 20 mm before detection.

D. MCA aneurysms are unique because they are more likely to present with IVH.

E. MCA aneurysms are unique because they are more likely to cause symptoms of mass effect than most other intracranial aneurysms.

✅ The answer is **D**.

— MCA aneurysms are unique because they are more likely to present with an ICH.

— The MCA is the third most common location of all intracranial aneurysms (about 20 %) and usually arises at the M1/M2 junction, projecting laterally in the plane of the M1 segment.

— They, by virtue of their angioarchitecture, are more challenging to treat with endovascular techniques than other aneurysms within the intracranial circulation.

❓ **92. MCA aneurysms**
Anatomy, the FALSE answer is:

A. Lying within the sylvian fissure, the MCA is the largest structure.

B. MCA has the most variable anatomy of the all intracranial arteries.

C. MCA is divided into five segments.

D. The M1 has multiple lenticulostriate arteries that are divided into medial and lateral lenticulostriate arteries.

E.   The medial lenticulostriate arteries supply the lentiform nucleus, the caudate, and the internal capsule.
F.   The lateral lenticulostriate arteries supply the caudate nucleus.

✅ The answer is **C**.
- MCA is divided into four segments: M1 (sphenoidal), M2 (insular), M3 (opercular), and M4 (cortical).
- The medial lenticulostriate arteries enter the anterior perforating substance superiorly and supply the lentiform nucleus, the caudate, and the internal capsule.
- The lateral lenticulostriate arteries are more variable in their location, traverse the basal ganglia, and supply the caudate nucleus.

❓ 93.   MCA aneurysms
Classification by morphology, the FALSE answer is:
A.   Saccular aneurysms are the most commonly encountered.
B.   Fusiform aneurysms can be encountered in MCA but less than saccular aneurysms.
C.   Blister aneurysms are more commonly described in the MCA distribution than on the ICA.
D.   Extremely dysmorphic or distal aneurysms are usually infectious and are classically identified on distal M4 branches.
E.   Bifurcation and trifurcation aneurysms represent up to 90 % of MCA aneurysms.

✅ The answer is **C**.
- Blister aneurysms are less commonly described in the MCA distribution than on the ICA.
- Bifurcation and trifurcation aneurysms represent up to 90 % of all MCA aneurysms and are the lesions most uniformly referred for surgical consideration.

❓ 94.   MCA aneurysms
Classification by morphology, the FALSE answer is:
A.   Aneurysms of the M1 segment are more common than bifurcation aneurysms.
B.   Proximal M1 segment lesions represent 2–12 % of all MCA aneurysms.
C.   In patients with multiple intracranial aneurysms, the frequency of proximal MCA aneurysms tends to increase.

D. Nearly three-fourths of patients with multiple intracranial aneurysms harbor an MCA aneurysm.

E. Distal MCA aneurysms are rare and can be either infectious or traumatic.

✅ The answer is **A**.

− Aneurysms of the M1 segment are second in frequency to bifurcation aneurysms and are composed of lenticulostriate or anterior temporal artery saccular aneurysms.

− Distal MCA aneurysms are the most uncommon of the MCA aneurysms and can be either infectious or, less frequently, traumatic. They also may require a modification of the traditional pterional approach or a different craniotomy entirely. By nature, they are often small and can be challenging to identify; stereotaxis may help facilitate their exposure. Treatment may require trapping and excision, vessel reconstruction, or extracranial intracranial bypass.

❓ 95. **MCA aneurysms**
   The FALSE answer is:
   A. Dissecting MCA aneurysms are rare and may be associated with infection.
   B. Traumatic MCA aneurysms are unusual and are most classically associated with a skull fracture.
   C. Traumatic MCA aneurysms have a high rupture rate.
   D. Traumatic MCA aneurysms are most frequently distal on M3 and M4 segments.
   E. Classically, traumatic MCA aneurysms are managed with endovascular coiling.

✅ The answer is **E**.

− Classically, traumatic MCA aneurysms are managed with surgical trapping and excision with or without bypass.

− Dissecting MCA aneurysms are rare and may be associated with infection, connective tissue diseases such as Marfan's syndrome, cystic medial degeneration, and fibromuscular dysplasia.

− Although most present with ischemia, 43 % of patients with an MCA aneurysmal dissection present with SAH, and 75 % of these patients are male.

− Traumatic MCA aneurysms are most frequently distal on M3 and M4 segments. And often present with delayed rupture (average, 4.7 days) after the inciting trauma.

96. MCA aneurysms
The FALSE answer is:
A. Cerebral aneurysms that reach large or giant size are more frequently seen in the MCA distribution than in other arterial distributions.
B. Giant MCA aneurysms represent up to 9 % of MCA aneurysms.
C. Giant MCA aneurysms may become symptomatic without SAH.
D. Giant aneurysms are reported to cause seizures more often than smaller ones.
E. Most M1-lenticulostriate aneurysms are usually giant size.

The answer is E.
- Most M1-lenticulostriate aneurysms are quite small (which often precludes endovascular treatment).
- Classification by size: aneurysms have been somewhat arbitrarily classified by size into small (<5 mm), medium (5–10 mm), large (11–25 mm), and giant (>25 mm).
- Giant aneurysms are reported to cause seizures more often than smaller ones, and this may be due to mass effect, ischemic changes, or repeated subclinical hemorrhages.

97. MCA aneurysms
Management, the FALSE answer is:
A. Typically, have large sacs containing intraluminal thrombus.
B. The intraluminal thrombus should be left in place without evacuation.
C. Giant aneurysms of the bifurcation that involve one or more of the branches may require vessel sacrifice with flow augmentation.
D. When performing the craniotomy preserve at least one branch of the STA.
E. If a low-flow bypass is anticipated preoperatively, the STA pedicle is dissected out with the opening.
F. High-flow extracranial-intracranial may be considered for fusiform aneurysms involving more than one branch.

The answer is B.
- Aneurysmorrhaphy: Typically, these large sacs contain intraluminal thrombus that must be removed before clip application. This requires temporary trapping and opening of the sac to evacuate the thrombus. An ultrasonic aspirator is often used to evacuate the intraluminal thrombus more rapidly to reduce temporary occlusion time.

- Bypass: Most MCA aneurysms can be safely clipped without difficulty and with minimal risk to the afferent or efferent vessels. However, fusiform and giant aneurysms of the bifurcation that involve one or more of the branches may require vessel sacrifice with flow augmentation to properly secure the aneurysm and perfuse the affected brain.
- When performing the craniotomy for all MCA aneurysms, we preserve at least one branch of the STA in the event an unanticipated STA-MCA bypass is needed.
- High-flow extracranial-intracranial bypasses using a saphenous vein or radial artery graft may need to be considered for fusiform aneurysms involving more than one branch when successful clip ligation is considered unlikely without it.

? 98. **MCA aneurysms**
   Approaches, the FALSE answer is:
   A. MCA aneurysms are preferentially clipped at most cerebrovascular centers.
   B. Proximal transsylvian approach carries more risk than distal transsylvian.
   C. Proximal transsylvian includes splitting the sylvian fissure medially and following the MCA trunk distally.
   D. Distal transsylvian includes following the major divisions proximally to the aneurysm by opening the fissure distally.
   E. Superior temporal gyrus (STG) approach: making a small corticotomy in the STG and then subsequently entering the distal portion of the sylvian fissure and following the M2 branches to the aneurysm.

✓ The answer is **B**.
- Proximal transsylvian approach is safer than distal transsylvian because of the early parent vessel control.

? 99. **Vertebral artery, PICA, and vertebro-basilar junction aneurysms**
   The FALSE answer is:
   A. Posterior circulation aneurysms (including PICA and basilar aneurysms) account for about 8–9 % of all intracranial aneurysms
   B. Non-PICA and basilar posterior circulation aneurysms account for 8 % of all intracranial aneurysms.
   C. These aneurysms can pose significant challenges because they arise at a region of the skull base.

D. These aneurysms can pose significant challenges because they occur in close proximity to the brainstem and lower cranial nerves.

E. These aneurysms can pose significant challenges because of the variability in the anatomy of the vertebral artery and PICA.

✅ The answer is **B**.

- Aneurysms from the proximal vertebral artery, the vertebral artery-PICA junction, the distal PICA, and the distal vertebral artery make up 25 % of all posterior circulation aneurysms and 2 % of all intracranial aneurysms.

❓ **100.** **Vertebral artery, PICA, and vertebro-basilar junction aneurysms The FALSE answer is:**

A. The incidence of fusiform aneurysms at the vertebro-basilar location, much more frequent than in the anterior circulation.

B. These aneurysms carry a high risk for rebleeding as well as high morbidity and mortality rates.

C. Fatal rebleeding in anterior circulation aneurysms is three times the number in the vertebro-basilar aneurysms.

D. Ruptured vertebral dissecting aneurysms carry a worse prognosis than saccular aneurysms of the same location.

E. Early surgical or endovascular treatment of the ruptured aneurysm is generally the rule.

✅ The answer is **C**.

- Fatal rebleeding in 10 % of vertebro-basilar aneurysms, three times the number in their anterior circulation aneurysm group.

- Vertebral dissections to account for 28 % of posterior circulation aneurysms with rebleeding rate from ruptured dissecting aneurysms has been reported to be 21–71 %.

❓ **101.** **Vertebral artery, PICA, and vertebro-basilar junction aneurysms The FALSE answer is:**

A. The most frequent clinical presentation of these aneurysms is SAH.

B. Unruptured aneurysms often present with signs and symptoms of ischemia or mass effect.

C. Angiography is the "gold standard" for diagnosis of vertebral dissection.

D. The vertebral dissection angiographic findings are string sign or rosette sign.

E. The vertebral dissection angiographic findings are pearl sign or double-lumen sign.

✅ The answer is **A**.
- The most frequent clinical presentation of these aneurysms is ICH.
- The vertebral dissection angiographic findings are string sign, rosette sign, pearl sign, tapered narrowing, occlusion, double lumen, or pseudoaneurysm.
- Suspicious cases of SAH in which no aneurysm or dissection is detected by CTA are followed up with a conventional four-vessel angiogram with rotational angiography and three-dimensional reconstructions as needed.

❓ 102. **Vertebral artery, PICA, and vertebro-basilar junction aneurysms (preoperative planning)**
The FALSE answer is:
   A. Should include careful attention to the presence of duplicated PICA
   B. Should include careful attention to the location of the ipsilateral PICA only
   C. Should include whether the PICA territory is supplied by an alternative vessel (such as the AICA)
   D. Should include to what degree the posterior cerebral arteries are being supplied through the posterior circulation
   E. Should include careful attention to the presence of fetal posterior cerebral arteries

✅ The answer is **B**.
- Should include careful attention to the location of both PICA and especially to the contralateral PICA

❓ 103. **Vertebral artery, PICA, and vertebro-basilar junction aneurysms***
   The FALSE answer is:
   A. For vertebral artery, PICA, and vertebro-basilar aneurysms, the most widely used are lateral suboccipital or far-lateral suboccipital approaches.
   B. Midline suboccipital or paramedian suboccipital approaches are used for more peripheral PICA aneurysms.
   C. For peripheral PICA aneurysms located in the tonsillomedullary segment, use the combined lateral and medial suboccipital approach.
   D. For PICA aneurysms in the segment distal to the cerebellotonsillar, use a standard midline suboccipital craniectomy extending through the foramen magnum.
   E. In far-lateral suboccipital approach, the preferred direction of approach is between the ninth (inferiorly) and the seventh and eighth cranial nerves (superiorly).

✓ The answer is **E**.
- In far-lateral suboccipital approach, the preferred direction of approach is in the space between the 11th inferiorly and the 9th and 10th cranial nerves superiorly.
- Most PICA aneurysms project **superiorly** according to Rhoton's third rule.
- Rhoton's third rule: Saccular aneurysms point in the direction that the blood would have gone if the curve at the aneurysm site were not present. The aneurysm dome or fundus points in the direction of the maximal hemodynamic thrust in the pre-aneurysmal segment of the parent artery.
- Tandem clipping is common with PICA aneurysms because the far-lateral approach provides a view along the axis of the VA, the aneurysms project superiorly, and the PICA often originates from the aneurysm base.
- In unusually high vertebro-basilar junction aneurysms, use the combined subtemporal-presigmoid transtentorial approach (the vertebro-basilar junction can be accessed by a window formed between the seventh and eighth nerves superiorly and the lower cranial nerves inferiorly).
- Treatment of vertebral dissecting and fusiform aneurysms: surgical treatments include proximal or parent artery occlusion (Hunterian ligation), trapping procedures, and clip reconstructions.
- Endovascular options include parent vessel occlusion, stent placement, and combinations of coil and stent therapies, in which the ipsilateral vertebral artery proximal to the aneurysm is occluded. This occlusion can be accomplished through a direct surgical approach by clipping the vertebral artery or by endovascular occlusions using balloons or coils.

❓ 104. **Basilar trunk aneurysms (BTA)**
   The FALSE answer is:
   A. BTAs are those located between the vertebro-basilar junction (VBJ) and the takeoff of the SCAs.
   B. The origin of AICA is a common site.
   C. More severe clinical sequelae are frequently observed after aneurysm rupture in this region.
   D. The severe clinical sequelae include syncope, coma, and death.
   E. The mortality rate associated with ruptured BTAs is around 0.3 %.

✓ The answer is **E**.
- The mortality rate associated with ruptured BTAs remains high, around 30 %.
- The origin of AICA is a common site for many of these aneurysms and is therefore also frequently referred to in order to distinguish upper BTAs (those located between AICA and SCA) from lower BTAs (those located between the AICA and VBJ).

105. Basilar trunk aneurysms
Presentation, the FALSE answer is:
A. Unruptured BTAs frequently present secondary to mass effect on brainstem and the related cranial nerves.
B. Usually aneurysms of the basilar apex, SCA, and upper basilar trunk may result in oculomotor nerve paresis.
C. Middle BTAs in the region of the AICA may result in abducent nerve paresis, facial nerve paresis, or hearing loss.
D. Those located at the VBJ may present secondary to mass effect on the fifth cranial nerve.
E. Signs of brainstem compression, such as hemiparesis, hemisensory deficits, and gait imbalance, may result from mass effect of unruptured BTAs.

The answer is **D**.
- Those located at the VBJ may present secondary to mass effect on the **9th, 10th, and 11th cranial** nerves.

106. Basilar trunk aneurysms
The FALSE answer is:
A. The mean length of the basilar artery is 30 mm.
B. The mean diameter of the basilar artery is 3–4 mm.
C. The size of the Pcom will not reflect the patient's ability to tolerate complete parent artery occlusion.
D. Complex or fusiform BTAs may not be amenable to clip ligation or direct aneurysm coiling.
E. Complex or fusiform BTAs may require endovascular occlusion of the parent basilar artery.

The answer is **C**.
- The size of the Pcom is an important prognostic factor in determining a patient's ability to tolerate complete parent artery occlusion.
- A balloon occlusion test is performed before complete occlusion, in which multiple modalities are used to demonstrate that the basilar artery can be safely occluded without evidence of brainstem ischemia.
- More recently, stent-assisted coiling for BTAs has been used.

107. Basilar trunk aneurysms
APPROACH selection, the FALSE answer is:
A. The relationship of the basilar apex to the foramen magnum is a major factor in the preoperative planning of such aneurysms.

B. Aneurysms <18 mm below sellar floor and small/medium sized favoring subtemporal transtentorial approach.

C. Midline aneurysms lying >18 mm below sellar floor or large aneurysms of basilar trunk or vertebro-basilar junction favoring combined supra-infratentorial (petrosal) approach.

D. Aneurysms lying >18 mm below sellar floor, small aneurysms of basilar trunk or vertebro-basilar junction and anteriorly arising tentorial origin of a dominant vein of Labbe on side of approach favoring lateral suboccipital or transcondylar approaches.

E. Subtemporal and petrosal (combined supra/infratentorial) approaches risk damage to the vein of Labbe.

✔ The answer is **A**.

━ The relationship of the basilar apex to the dorsum sella is a major factor in the preoperative planning of such aneurysms.

❓ 108. **Basilar trunk aneurysms***
APPROACH selection, the FALSE answer is:

A. Upper BTAs can be treated with a standard pterional or OZ approach.

B. The transoral-transclival approach has also been used to treat aneurysms of the lower basilar trunk and VBJ.

C. The transoral-transclival approach carries a great risk of transtentorial herniation.

D. Temporary proximal balloon occlusion offers the benefits of proximal control before initiation of the exposure.

E. Balloon occlusion may be used as a transient measure to test whether the basilar artery can be permanently occluded.

✔ The answer is **C**.

━ The transoral-transclival approach has also been used to treat aneurysms of the lower basilar trunk and VBJ, yet carries a great risk of CSF leak and meningitis.

━ Temporary proximal balloon occlusion offers the benefits of proximal control before initiation of the exposure, avoidance of obstruction of the operative field by the temporary clip, and ability to confirm occlusion of the aneurysm sac with digital subtraction angiography.

━ Endovascular balloon occlusion testing can be used in conjunction with neuroleptic anesthesia, SPECT imaging, and neurophysiologic monitoring to determine the safety and feasibility of a planned complete occlusion.

? 109. **Basilar apex (bifurcation) (tip) aneurysms**
   The FALSE answer is:
   A. Basilar apex account for about half of posterior circulation aneurysms.
   B. In basilar apex, the more posterior the aneurysm, the poorer the prognosis.
   C. The interpeduncular cistern is enclosed by clivus and posterior clinoid process anteriorly, medial aspects of temporal lobes, and tentorium laterally.
   D. Membrane of Liliequist forms posterior boundary of interpeduncular cistern.
   E. The interpeduncular cistern is enclosed by the cerebral peduncles posteriorly, and the mammillary bodies and posterior perforated substance superiorly.

✓ The answer is **D**.
   − Membrane of Liliequist forms an anterior "curtain" for the interpeduncular cistern. This membrane is a thick layer of arachnoid that anchors from the mammillary bodies superiorly and extends anteriorly and inferiorly before folding posteriorly to form the roof of the prepontine cistern.
   − In basilar bifurcation aneurysms, the more posterior the aneurysm, the poorer the prognosis, because the tendency for vital perforators to be involved becomes greater as the aneurysm projects more posteriorly.

? 110. **Basilar apex aneurysms**
   The FALSE answer is:
   A. The terminal basilar artery lies about 15 mm posterior to the posterior aspect of the ICAs.
   B. Basilar apex can be located above, below, or at the level of the dorsum sellae.
   C. The size of the P1 segment of the PCA depends on the extent to which the Pcom contributes to blood flow in the distal PCA.
   D. The cranial nerve most intimately associated with basilar apex aneurysms is the trochlear nerve.
   E. Preservation of the posterior thalamoperforating arteries is an essential technical nuance of basilar apex aneurysm surgery.

✅ The answer is **D**.
  - The cranial nerve most intimately associated with basilar apex aneurysms is the oculomotor nerve that traverses the space between the PCA and the SCA within the interpeduncular cistern.
  - The size of the segment of the PCA from the basilar bifurcation to the junction with the Pcom (P1) depends on the extent to which the Pcom contributes to blood flow in the distal PCA. A fetal PCA implies that the P1 is a vestigial band, with all PCA blood flow originating from the carotid artery.
  - Preservation of the thalamoperforating arteries is an essential technical nuance of basilar apex aneurysm surgery. These critical perforators arise from the posterior aspect of the basilar trunk, the proximal P1 segments, and the posterior communicating arteries.

❓ 111. **Basilar apex aneurysms**
       Approach, the FALSE answer is:
       A. The two pure approaches for basilar apex aneurysms are the subtemporal approach and the transsylvian approach.
       B. Fundus pointing posteriorly and low basilar bifurcation are favoring subtemporal approach.
       C. High basilar bifurcation and narrow neck are favoring transsylvian approach.
       D. The presence of other anterior circulation aneurysms on the side of approach is favoring transsylvian pterional approach.
       E. In pure transsylvian approach, proximal control is very complicated.

✅ The answer is **E**.
  - In pure transsylvian approach, proximal control is straightforward.
  - Also see comments on the next question.

❓ 112. **Basilar apex aneurysms**
       Subtemporal approach, the FALSE answer is:
       A. Offers proximal control is easy.
       B. The lateral view facilitates dissection of the perforators.
       C. Exposure and clipping of anteriorly or posteriorly directed aneurysms are more feasible than with the transsylvian approach.
       D. The field is very wide.
       E. Intraoperative bleeding can be difficult to control.

✔️ The answer is **D**. The field is narrow.

— **The pure transsylvian approach has several assets:**
1. Neurosurgeons are familiar with this approach because it is used for more common aneurysms and tumors.
2. Proximal control is straightforward.
3. Exposure of both P1 segments for temporary trapping is uncomplicated.
4. Wide exposure is possible.

— **The transsylvian exposure also has liabilities:**
1. Exposure of posteriorly located perforators is difficult.
2. Inspection of distal aspect of clip blade is difficult.
3. Technical features make treatment of directly anteriorly or directly posteriorly projecting aneurysms very difficult.

— **The subtemporal approach offers the surgeon many assets:**
1. Proximal control is easy.
2. The lateral view facilitates dissection of the perforators.
3. Tentorial division allows exposure of the upper one-third of the clivus for low-lying bifurcations.
4. Fenestrated clips can be placed with excellent visualization of the thalamoperforators.
5. Exposure and clipping of anteriorly or posteriorly directed aneurysms are more feasible than with the transsylvian.

— **The subtemporal exposure also has liabilities:**
1. The field is narrow.
2. Access to the proximal contralateral P1 for temporary trapping is poor.
3. The temporal lobe can be injured in fresh SAH in poor-grade or obese patients.
4. Cranial nerve III palsy often occurs postoperatively (usually transient).
5. Intraoperative bleeding can be difficult to control.

❓ 113. **Basilar apex aneurysms**
   Pterional approach, the TRUE answer is:
   A. PAVEL means pterional approach via the extended lateral corridor.
   B. Lateral dissection plane and clipping are better from the surgeon's dominant side.
   C. If patient has right hemiparesis or left oculomotor palsy, the approach must be from the right side.
   D. The surgical field is centered on cranial nerve III.
   E. Risks include oculomotor palsy in 30 % which is usually temporary.

✔ The answer is **C.**
- If patient has right hemiparesis or left oculomotor palsy, the approach must be from the left side.
- Pterional approach via the extended lateral corridor (PAVEL)
- The essential elements of PAVEL include the following:
  1. It is performed from the surgeon's dominant side, which facilitates a due lateral dissection plane and clipping.
  2. Wide opening of the sylvian fissure is possible.
  3. The surgical field is centered on cranial nerve III.
  4. Mesial temporal lobe structures are elevated out of the incisura to the level of the cerebral peduncle.
  5. Posterior dissection is performed behind and below ipsilateral P1, not through the neck.
  6. The initial clip is fenestrated with a very small blade to close the contralateral neck.
  7. The final clip is a short, conventional clip to eliminate residual neck filling through the fenestration.
- Pterional approach is from the right unless:
  1. Additional left-sided aneurysm (e.g., Pcom aneurysm) which could be treated simultaneously by a left-sided approach.
  2. Aneurysm points to the right.
  3. Aneurysm is located to the left of midline (the operation is more difficult when the aneurysm is even just 2–3 mm contralateral to the craniotomy).
  4. Patient has right hemiparesis or left oculomotor palsy.

❓ 114. **Basilar apex aneurysms**
   TIMING OF TREATMENT, the FALSE answer is:
   A. The peak incidence of repeat hemorrhage after SAH occurs in the first 48 h.
   B. Early surgery after SAH avoids the morbidity and mortality associated with repeat hemorrhage.
   C. It has been better to do early surgery in the high-grade Hunt and Hess patient.
   D. Frequently endovascular treatment is considered for patients with high clinical grades.
   E. Of the various approaches, the subtemporal approach is particularly not well tolerated soon after hemorrhage in the high-grade patient.

✔️ The answer is **C**.
- It has been better to **delay surgery in the high-grade patient** (i.e., Hunt and Hess grades IV and V) for a few days unless acceptable occlusion with endovascular therapy is feasible.
- The peak incidence of vasospasm occurs 7–10 days after SAH.
- Early surgery after SAH avoids the morbidity and mortality associated with repeat hemorrhage and allows aggressive medical and interventional management of vasospasm. However, certain patients with basilar apex aneurysms may be harmed by early surgery.
- Occasionally aminocaproic acid is used in patients for whom we delay surgery, particularly if the subarachnoid portion of the bleeding is modest.
- Proximal occlusion and trapping have important roles in basilar apex aneurysm surgery.
- To achieve complete aneurysm occlusion safely in a high percentage of patients, coiling should be limited to small aneurysms with neck sizes less than 4 mm and PCAs that do not originate from the dome.

❓ **115. Intracranial aneurysms**
   Endovascular approaches, the FALSE answer is:
   A. Balloon remodeling is more often used to Pcom than for Acom aneurysms.
   B. Coiling remains the endovascular treatment of choice for MCA aneurysms.
   C. Inferiorly and posteriorly projecting Acom are more difficult to coil.
   D. Difficult coiling is usually due to suboptimal visualization and catheter instability within the aneurysm.
   E. Pericallosal aneurysms are frequently amenable to coil embolization.

✔️ The answer is **B**.
- Coiling remains the endovascular treatment of choice for Acom aneurysms.

❓ **116. Intracranial aneurysms**
   Endovascular approaches, the FALSE answer is:
   A. Once the anatomic characteristics of the Pcom have been delineated, coil embolization of these lesions is typically straightforward.
   B. Unlike Pcom, ophthalmic aneurysms are difficult to be managed through endovascular techniques.

C. Cavernous aneurysms treated by detachable balloon embolization of the aneurysm and later by the advent of aneurysm coiling.
D. MCA aneurysm particularly challenging for endovascular treatment.
E. The relatively small caliber of the MCA compared with the proximal ICA increases the risk of complications.

✅ The answer is **B**.
- Like Pcom aneurysms, ophthalmic aneurysms are **easily** managed through endovascular techniques.
- MCA aneurysm particularly challenging for endovascular treatment. Compromise of any of the MCA branches by the coil mass risks a devastating ischemic or thromboembolic insult.

❓ 117. **Intracranial aneurysms***
Endovascular approaches, the FALSE answer is:
A. Balloon remodeling of PICA is challenging.
B. Balloon remodeling of PICA may require trans-circulation navigation of the balloon from the contralateral vertebral artery.
C. Endovascular techniques are not suited for treatment of PICA aneurysms.
D. Treatment of choice for PCA is endovascular embolization.
E. Balloon and stent-assisted techniques are often mandatory for the treatment of PCA aneurysms.

✅ The answer is **C**.
- Endovascular techniques are ideally suited for the treatment of PICA aneurysms, which are difficult to approach surgically.
- Because of the difficulty of directly approaching PCA aneurysms microsurgically, the treatment of choice is endovascular embolization.

❓ 118. **Intracranial aneurysms***
Endovascular stenting, the FALSE answer is:
A. The basic principles underlying stent-supported aneurysm therapy are parent vessel protection and parent vessel remodeling.
B. Parent vessel protection prevents coil embolization.
C. Parent vessel remodeling includes stents that produce flow diversion and provide scaffolding for neo-intimal overgrowth.
D. Parent vessel remodeling may facilitate and maintain aneurysm thrombosis.
E. Parent vessel remodeling includes parent vessel configuration, flow redirection, and tissue overgrowth.

✔ The answer is **B**.

- Basic principles underlying stent-supported aneurysm therapy:
  1. Parent vessel protection: stents could be applied to provide durable parent vessel protection, facilitating the coil embolization of wide-necked aneurysms by preventing coil prolapse into the parent vessel.
  2. Parent vessel remodeling:
     A. Parent vessel configuration: The implantation of a stent within a parent artery may straighten the vessel, altering (possibly in a favorable manner) the flow dynamics within the aneurysm. The magnitude of this effect is affected primarily by the rigidity of the stent.
     B. Flow redirection: The presence of stent tines over the aneurysm neck functions to disrupt the inflow jet, reducing vortices and shear stress on the aneurysm wall and reducing the "water-hammer" effect of chronic pulsatile blood flow on an intra-aneurysmal coil mass. The magnitude of this is affected primarily by the amount of metal surface area coverage provided by the stent.
     C. Tissue overgrowth: the presence of a stent across the neck of the aneurysm provides a scaffolding and stimulus for the overgrowth of endothelial and neo-intimal tissue across the neck of the aneurysm, creating a "biologic remodeling" in the region of the aneurysm neck.

❓ 119. **Intracranial aneurysms***
Endosaccular packing include, FALSE answer is:
A. Endosaccular coil embolization.
B. Balloon-assisted coil embolization.
C. Endosaccular liquid embolic agents.
D. Neck bridge devices.
E. Flow diverters are not included.

✔ The answer is **E**.

- Endosaccular packing includes stent and coils or stent alone (flow diverter).

❓ 120. **Intracranial aneurysms**
Recurrence after endovascular treatment, the FALSE answer is:
A. Neck width >4 mm increases the risk of recurrence.
B. Overall sac size (small < large).
C. Presence of intra-saccular thrombus increases the risk of recurrence.
D. Recurrence rate is 60 % in large/giant dysplastic aneurysms.
E. Recurrence rate is more in small aneurysms with small neck.

✅ The answer is **E**.
  - The main factor influencing recurrence after endovascular treatment is the aneurysm sac and neck size.
  - Recurrence rates are 5–10 % in small aneurysms (<10 mm) with small necks (<4 mm), 20 % in small aneurysms with large necks, and 60 % in large/giant dysplastic aneurysms.

❓ 121. **Treatment of aneurysmal rupture during coiling**
  The FALSE answer is:
  A. Inflate balloon if balloon-assisted coiling is used.
  B. Immediately reverse anticoagulation.
  C. Stop packing coils as rapidly as possible.
  D. Continue to pack coils as rapidly as possible.
  E. Insert an extraventricular drain (EVD).

✅ The answer is **C**.
  - Immediately reverse anticoagulation (protamine should be available during the procedure).

❓ 122. **Intracranial aneurysms**
  Endovascular Hunterian ligation, the FALSE answer is:
  A. One of the oldest successful interventions for arterial aneurysms.
  B. Is permanent sacrifice of parent artery to prevent blood access to aneurysm.
  C. This technique has also been referred to as "reconstructive" therapy.
  D. Hunterian ligation most often targets complex aneurysms.
  E. Hunterian ligation can be used occasionally for vascular tumors.

✅ The answer is **C**.
  - This technique has also been referred to as "deconstructive" therapy, in contrast to "reconstructive" therapy, which refers to the targeted occlusion of a vascular abnormality without impairment of blood flow in the parent vessel.
  - One of the oldest successful interventions for arterial aneurysms— ligation of the femoral artery to treat a popliteal aneurysm by John Hunter in 1785.
  - The carotid arteries were the first cerebral vessels to be intentionally and successfully ligated in 1808 by the English surgeon Astley Cooper.
  - Hunterian ligation can be used occasionally for hemorrhagic stroke, vascular tumors, arteriovenous malformations, fistulas, and arterial dissections.

? 123. Intracranial aneurysms*
Endovascular approaches (INDICATIONS), the FALSE answer is:
A. Hunterian ligation is reserved primarily for giant and fusiform aneurysms.
B. Some traumatic aneurysms may be candidates.
C. Some infectious aneurysms may be candidates.
D. The current standard of care requires preoperative evaluation with balloon test occlusion.
E. Occlusion of the vertebral artery was most effective at its origin from subclavian artery.

✔ The answer is **E**.
— Occlusion of the vertebral artery was most effective at the level of C1 because antegrade collateral flow is possible through the external carotid artery.
— The current standard of care requires preoperative evaluation with balloon test occlusion (BTO) followed by distal perfusion.
— The major treatment question when considering endovascular Hunterian ligation is whether to perform an arterial bypass before permanent vessel occlusion.

? 124. PICA aneurysms*
Endovascular approaches, the FALSE answer is:
A. If aneurysm is separated from the origin of PICA, internal occlusion is done.
B. If aneurysm involves the origin of PICA and has SAH, proximal occlusion and internal trapping is preferred.
C. If aneurysm involves the origin of PICA and has no SAH, direct internal occlusion is done.
D. If aneurysm involves the origin of PICA and has no SAH, BTO followed by occipital artery-PICA bypass is preferred.
E. Too much collateral flow can prevent aneurysmal thrombosis.

✔ The answer is **C**.

? 125. Intracranial aneurysms
Complications of endovascular approaches, the FALSE answer is:
A. Ischemic stroke
B. Post-occlusion thromboembolism
C. Coil migration
D. Secondary AVM development
E. Perforator occlusion

✅ The answer is **D**.
- ━ Secondary aneurysm development

❓ **126. Giant intracranial aneurysms**
The FALSE answer is:
A. Giant aneurysms represent 2–5 % of all intracranial aneurysms.
B. Giant intracranial aneurysms have a minimum diameter of at least 25 mm.
C. Giant aneurysms have a male preponderance.
D. Most patients become symptomatic in the fourth through sixth decades of life.
E. Giant aneurysms currently remain primarily a surgical disease.

✅ The answer is **C**.
- ━ As with other aneurysms, giant aneurysms have a female preponderance.
- ━ Giant aneurysms currently remain primarily a surgical disease that must be managed effectively to minimize morbidity.

❓ **127. Giant intracranial aneurysms**
The FALSE answer is:
A. Giant aneurysms are found in ACA mainly.
B. Giant aneurysms may result directly from trauma.
C. More than one aneurysm may be present in 10–36 % of patients.
D. A significant proportion of giant aneurysms have associated intraluminal thrombus.
E. The presence of a partially thrombosed aneurysm does not appear to lower the risk for rupture of the aneurysm.

✅ The answer is **A**.
- ━ In general, 34–67 % of giant intracranial aneurysms are associated with the ICA, 11–40 % with the anterior cerebral artery and middle cerebral artery (MCA), and 13–56 % with the vertebral and basilar arteries.
- ━ A significant proportion of giant aneurysms have associated intraluminal thrombosis—as many as 60 % in some series.

❓ **128. Giant intracranial aneurysms**
Presentation, the FALSE answer is:
A. Signs and symptoms due to a mass effect develop in approximately two-thirds.
B. Only about a third of patients have SAH as the initial symptom.

C. 7 % of patients with giant aneurysms initially had ischemic symptoms.
D. Annual rupture rate for giant aneurysms is lower than small aneurysms.
E. Annual rupture rate for giant intracranial aneurysms of around 6 %.

✓ The answer is **D**.
- Annual rupture rate for giant intracranial aneurysms of around 6 %, higher than the 1–3 % rate quoted for smaller aneurysms.

❓ 129. **Giant intracranial aneurysms**
Management, the FALSE answer is:
A. The approaches used for giant aneurysms of the posterior fossa include orbitozygomatic, transpetrosal, or far-lateral approaches.
B. Circulatory arrest permits complete vascular control, but increase the risk for intraoperative rupture of the aneurysm.
C. Hypothermic circulatory arrest can facilitate the surgical technique.
D. The absence of blood flow greatly facilitates clip reconstruction.
E. Endovascular techniques are more preferred for giant cavernous sinus aneurysms.

✓ The answer is **B**.
- Circulatory arrest permits complete vascular control and the risk for intraoperative rupture of the aneurysm is eliminated.
- Hypothermic circulatory arrest can facilitate the surgical technique by allowing more aggressive manipulation of the aneurysm dome without fear of rupture.

❓ 130. **Giant intracranial aneurysms**
Hypothermic circulatory arrest, the FALSE answer is:
A. Deep hypothermia increases the brain's metabolic requirements for oxygen.
B. During circulatory arrest, adequate cerebral protection with barbiturates is imperative.
C. Hypothermic circulatory arrest is associated with a mortality rate of 8 %.
D. The risks related to hypothermic circulatory arrest include coagulopathies.
E. The risks related to hypothermic circulatory arrest include hemodilution after blood products and intravenous fluids are replaced.

✔ The answer is **A**.
— Deep hypothermia reduces the brain's metabolic requirements for oxygen.
— Hypothermic arrest associated with 13 % morbidity and 8 % mortality.

❓ **131. Giant intracranial aneurysms**
Surgical requirements, the FALSE answer is:
A. A comparatively larger craniotomy flap
B. Extremely lax brain
C. Restricted exposure of the sylvian cistern
D. Wide roomy exposure of the sylvian cistern
E. Satisfactory exposure of surrounded arteries for temporary occlusion

✔ The answer is **C**.

❓ **132. Infectious intracranial aneurysms**
The FALSE answer is:
A. Mycotic aneurysms came to describe all aneurysms of infectious origin.
B. Intracranial aneurysms of infectious etiology are rare and represent approximately 2–6 % of all intracranial aneurysms.
C. The incidence may be higher in children.
D. Fungal or "true" mycotic aneurysms are rare.
E. The incidence of these lesions has recently decreased.

✔ The answer is **E**.
— Fungal or "true" mycotic aneurysms are rare. However, the incidence of these lesions has recently increased as a result of more patients with immunocompromised states.
— The incidence may be higher in children, in whom they account for as many as 10 % of all intracranial aneurysms.

❓ **133. Infectious intracranial aneurysms**
The FALSE answer is:
A. These are typically friable lesions.
B. Can be divided into intravascular and extravascular origin of infection.
C. These from extravascular source such as meningitis tend to occur proximally.

D. These from extravascular source such as meningitis tend to occur distally.

E. Embolic infectious aneurysms associated with infective endocarditis occur predominantly in distal cerebral arterial regions.

✅ The answer is **D**.
- These are typically friable lesions and often not separable from the surrounding parenchyma, which plays an important role in surgical planning.

❓ **134. Infectious intracranial aneurysms**
Intravascular infection, the FALSE answer is:
A. Intravascularly infectious aneurysms are bacterial but may rarely be fungal.
B. Intravascularly infectious aneurysms tend to form in branch points in the distal vasculature.
C. The most common location is the DACA.
D. Infectious aneurysms are most commonly from mitral valve septic vegetations.
E. Numerous emboli cause multiple aneurysms in as many as 30 % of patients.

✅ The answer is **E**.
- The most common location is the distal MCA.
- Because of their embolic etiology, intravascularly derived infectious aneurysms tend to form in locations where blood flow is maximal, and the vascular anatomy favors the lodging of embolic particles, such as vessel branch points in the distal vasculature.
- This contrasts with classic berry aneurysms, which tend to form on large basal vessels as solitary lesions.
- The most common location is the distal MCA, where more than 60 % of emboli lodge.

❓ **135. Infectious intracranial aneurysms**
The FALSE answer is:
A. Endocarditis, particularly left-sided valve disease, predisposes patient to infectious aneurysms and neurological complications.
B. 80 % of intracranial infectious aneurysms are due to endocarditis.
C. 20–40 % of patients with endocarditis suffer neurological sequelae.
D. Cerebral infarction is the least common.
E. Intracranial hemorrhage occurs in 5 %.

✅ The answer is **D**.
- Cerebral infarction is most common and affects up to 31 % of patients.
- Overall, in 1–4 % of patients with infective endocarditis, an infectious intracranial aneurysm is clinically diagnosed.

❓ **136.** **Infectious intracranial aneurysms (extravascular)**
   The FALSE answer is:
   A. Extravascular infection can extend into the arterial wall and induce arteritis.
   B. The most common location for extravascular infection is the MCA.
   C. *Streptococcus viridans* and *Staphylococcus aureus* are most common.
   D. Multiple organisms are found in less than 5 % of patients.
   E. Despite multiple blood or CSF cultures, 20 % fail to grow an organism.

✅ The answer is **B**.
- Usual locations include the intracavernous ICA, the midbasilar artery, and the vertebral artery.
- Extravascular infection such as meningitis can potentially extend into the arterial wall and induce arteritis and aneurysm formation.
- Extravascular infection such as meningitis, cavernous sinus thrombophlebitis, cerebral abscess, subdural empyema, osteomyelitis of the skull, tonsillitis, pharyngitis, sinusitis, and wound infection, as well as drug abuse, can potentially extend into the arterial wall and induce arteritis and aneurysm formation.
- *Streptococcus viridans* and *Staphylococcus aureus* are responsible for 57–90 % of infectious intracranial aneurysms.
- Despite multiple blood or CSF cultures, at least 12–20 % of patients fail to grow an organism.

❓ **137.** **Infectious intracranial aneurysms**
   FUNGAL, the FALSE answer is:
   A. Most fungal aneurysms find their origin in the extravascular space.
   B. These "true" mycotic aneurysms are smaller and more saccular in shape.
   C. *Aspergillus* is the most common fungus cultured.
   D. The tendency of *Aspergillus* for intramural growth is directly related to the fusiform shape seen with fungal aneurysms.
   E. Aspergillosis of the CNS is usually from direct infection of paranasal sinuses.

✅ The answer is **B**.

- These "true" mycotic aneurysms tend to be larger and more fusiform in shape with a higher association of occlusion of the vessel than occurs with bacterial aneurysms.
- *Aspergillus* is the most common fungus cultured, followed by Phycomycetes and *Candida albicans*.
- Aneurysms of fungal etiology usually occur in immunocompromised hosts.
- Direct spread of a fungal infection associated with an aneurysm after craniofacial and other neurosurgical procedures has also been described.
- Aspergillosis of the CNS is usually from direct infection via the paranasal sinus or indirectly by hematogenous spread (lungs).

❓ 138. **Infectious intracranial aneurysms**
The FALSE answer is:
A. The most common manifestation is a focal neurological deficit.
B. Focal neurological deficit occurred in about 50 % of patients.
C. Majority of neurological manifestations in patients with endocarditis are due to an infectious aneurysm.
D. Rheumatic heart disease and related valvular abnormalities are important predisposing factor.
E. Prosthetic valves and intravenous drug abuse have become important predisposing factors.

✅ The answer is **C**.

- Neurological manifestations are common in patients with endocarditis, with only a minority ultimately referable to an infectious aneurysm.
- The most common manifestation is a focal neurological deficit, which occurred in 48 % of patients in one larger series. This finding is in contrast to other intracranial aneurysms, which are much less likely to be accompanied by focal signs or symptoms.
- Prosthetic valves, elderly sclerotic valve disease, and nosocomially acquired bloodstream infections and intravenous drug abuse have become the most important predisposing factors.

❓ 139. **Infectious intracranial aneurysms**
The FALSE answer is:
A. The mortality associated with infectious aneurysms is highly variable, ranging from 12 % to as high as 80 %.
B. Most important prognostic factor for outcome is the presence of ischemia.

C. Intracranial hemorrhage in the setting of endocarditis is a strong indication for cerebral angiography.
D. Intracranial fungal aneurysms impart an even worse prognosis.
E. Intracranial fungal aneurysms mortality rate is greater than 90 % despite medical or surgical therapy.

✅ The answer is **B**.
- The most important prognostic factor for outcome is the presence of hemorrhage.
- CSF cultures in patients with intracranial aneurysms of infectious etiology will often fail to grow an organism, with one study finding CSF cultures positive in just 16 % of patients.

❓ **140.** **Infectious intracranial aneurysms**
Indications for conservative management, the FALSE answer is:
A. Unruptured aneurysms.
B. Aneurysm arising from the proximal cerebral vessels and sacrifice of the parent artery is not possible.
C. Surgical obliteration of aneurysms results in serious neurological deficits.
D. Progression of aneurysms while undergoing antibiotic therapy.
E. Fungal aneurysms.

✅ The answer is **D**.
- Regression of aneurysms while undergoing antibiotic therapy.
- Neurological complications can develop in up to 30 % of patients after the initiation of antibiotic therapy.
- Consequently, follow-up angiography is important to monitor intracranial infectious aneurysms during antibiotic treatment, and aneurysmal growth should prompt urgent surgical treatment.

❓ **141.** **Infectious intracranial aneurysms**
Indications for surgical intervention, the FALSE answer is:
A. The presence of symptomatic mass effect from a hematoma or the aneurysm
B. An unruptured aneurysm
C. Enlargement of an aneurysm during appropriate antibiotic treatment
D. Failure of an aneurysm to resolve despite a full course of appropriate antibiotic therapy
E. Neurological deterioration during antibiotic therapy

✅ The answer is **B**. Ruptured aneurysm

❓ 142. **Infectious intracranial aneurysms***
The FALSE answer is:
A. Whenever possible, a short course of antibiotics should be given to allow reparative fibrosis of the aneurysm.
B. Clipping is very effective if the aneurysm is friable in nature and adherence to surrounding parenchyma.
C. Excision of the aneurysm with a short segment of parent vessel is a potent treatment option but can be performed only in distal non-eloquent vessel.
D. In patients who cannot tolerate endovascular occlusion of the parent vessel, surgery should be planned.
E. In those patients, surgical options include potential bypass, reanastomosis, or sparing of the parent artery.

✅ The answer is **B**.
– Clipping is frequently not possible if the aneurysm is friable nature and adherence to surrounding parenchyma.

❓ 143. **Neoplastic intracranial aneurysms***
The FALSE answer is:
A. The classic cause is cardiac myxoma.
B. Cardiac myxoma usually involves the left atrium and tumor emboli are carried to cranial arteries.
C. The commonest site is the ICA.
D. Metastatic choriocarcinoma may also cause aneurysms.
E. Rarely, local spread by tumors at the skull base and invasion of the arterial wall causes an aneurysm.

✅ The answer is **C**.
– The commonest sites are branches of the MCA, and aneurysms are either fusiform or saccular in shape and often multiple.
– A rare type of aneurysm is usually caused by intravascular metastasis rather than arterial wall invasion by tumor.
– Metastatic choriocarcinoma may also invade intracranial arteries and cause arterial rupture, occlusion, or aneurysms by disrupting the internal elastic laminar and media.

144. Multiple intracranial aneurysms
The FALSE answer is:
A. Incidence of multiple aneurysms is 15–20 %.
B. In patients with multiple aneurysms, the most common site is DACA.
C. In patients with multiple aneurysms, the second most common site is MCA.
D. Bilateral symmetrical aneurysms (mirror aneurysms) may occur.
E. In the setting of an aneurysmal SAH, the risk for subsequent rupture of additional incidental aneurysms is significantly higher.

✓ The answer is **B**.
— In patients with multiple aneurysms, the most common sites are ICA and MCA.

145. Multiple intracranial aneurysms
Risk factors, the FALSE answer is:
A. Hypertension, smoking, and female gender (especially postmenopausal women) are significant risk factors.
B. Sickle cell disease.
C. Polycystic kidney disease, Ehlers-Danlos syndrome, and Marfan's syndrome.
D. 1 % of AVM-associated aneurysms are multiple.
E. Patients with familial aneurysms and multiple aneurysms tend to be younger.

✓ The answer is **D**.
— 40–50 % of AVM-associated aneurysms are multiple. Most of these aneurysms being located on the feeding vessel of the AVM (85 %).
— Hypertension found to be most important one associated with multiplicity.
— Patients with familial aneurysms and multiple aneurysms tend to be younger, and there is a higher incidence of MCA and ICA.
— 57 % of sickle cell disease had more than one aneurysm.
— Rare cases of hereditary connective tissue diseases, such as polycystic kidney disease, Ehlers-Danlos syndrome, pseudoxanthoma elasticum, and Marfan's syndrome are also risk factors.

? 146. Multiple intracranial aneurysms*
Prediction of rupture site:
When a patient present with SAH and is found to have multiple aneurysms, the following may be clues as to which aneurysm has bled; the FALSE answer is:

A. Epicenter (center of greatest concentration) of blood on CT or MRI.
B. In MRI, focal edema or increased signal adjacent to one aneurysm may indicate a recent hemorrhage.
C. In angiography, aneurysm bleb, irregular contour ("Murphy's tit") signs.
D. Focal vasospasm, changing aneurysm shape in serial angiograms, and extravasation of contrast.
E. If none of the above help, then suspect the smallest aneurysm is the source.

✓ The answer is **E**.
- If none of the above help, then suspect the largest aneurysm is the source.
- Other assisting points: history, clinical exam, EEG, and isotope scan (rapid flow suggests perfusion; static flow suggests infarct).
- False localization of the ruptured site may result in disastrous postoperative hemorrhage from the unprotected ruptured aneurysm.
- The most common cause of post-op bleeding was felt to be from rebleeding of the original aneurysm which ruptured that was missed on initial angiogram.

? 147. Revascularization techniques for complex aneurysms
The FALSE answer is:

A. Indicated if atherosclerosis of the aneurysm neck or the parent artery can make clipping dangerous or impossible.
B. Indicated if recurrent aneurysms after endovascular coil embolization may be unclippable.
C. Treatment options include clip occlusion of the aneurysm along with the branching vessel or vessels, parent artery Hunterian ligation, and trapping.
D. All proximal vessel occlusion often results in ischemia, and therefore bypass should be considered.
E. Even if the patient passes a balloon test occlusion, there remains up to a 20 % chance of stroke with complete occlusion without a bypass.

✅ The answer is **D**.

- Proximal vessel occlusion (ICA or vertebral artery) **may be tolerated without bypass.**
- Occlusion of branches such as the MCA, AICA, and PICA often result in ischemia, and therefore bypass should be considered.
- Preoperative evaluation by angiography and balloon test occlusion (with or without hypotensive provocative testing or cerebral blood flow measurements) may aid in the identification of patients who can tolerate carotid sacrifice.

❓ **148.** **Revascularization procedures for complex aneurysms**
   Bypass types, the FALSE answer is:
   A. Type I bypass: interposition vein grafts
   B. Type II bypass: extracranial-to-intracranial bypass with a saphenous vein or radial artery graft
   C. Type III bypass: scalp artery (STA or occipital) extracranial-to-intracranial bypass
   D. Type IV bypass: extracranial-to-intracranial bypass
   E. Type IV bypass: direct intracranial revascularization

✅ The answer is **D**.

❓ **149.** **Revascularization procedures for complex aneurysms***
   Type I bypass, the FALSE answer is:
   A. Type I bypass involves an interposition graft from the parent artery proximal to the site of occlusion to the point immediately distal to the parent artery.
   B. The primary example is the purely intracranial petrous carotid-to-supraclinoid carotid saphenous vein interposition graft.
   C. The most important disadvantage is that it requires prolonged occlusion of ECA.
   D. Being technically complex and requiring a lengthy procedure are also disadvantages.
   E. It is associated with a significant complication rate related to graft occlusion and perioperative ischemic brain injury.

✅ The answer is **C**.

- The most important disadvantage is that it requires a prolonged period of ICA occlusion.

? 150. **Revascularization procedures for complex aneurysms***
Type II bypass, the FALSE answer is:
A. Type II bypass consists of a saphenous vein interposition graft between the extracranial carotid artery and a major intracranial branch vessel.
B. This procedure is used when major arterial trunk must be occluded to treat tumor or giant aneurysm and distal collateral circulation is inadequate.
C. A vein graft generally has higher long-term patency.
D. A vein graft has higher risk of kinking and caliber mismatch.
E. A type II bypass can be a substitute for an STA-MCA bypass when the scalp artery is hypoplastic or occluded.

✅ The answer is **C**.
- A vein graft generally has lower long-term patency, higher risk of kinking, and caliber mismatch between the larger vein and smaller intracranial vessels.
- Type II bypasses: extracranial-to-intracranial bypass with a saphenous vein graft or radial artery graft.

? 151. **Revascularization procedures for complex aneurysms***
Type III bypass, the FALSE answer is:
A. Is extracranial-to-intracranial bypass via scalp artery (superficial temporal or occipital).
B. This procedure is performed when a giant aneurysm requires occlusion of a single, crucial arterial branch.
C. This procedure is performed when carotid occlusion is required and the circle of Willis is only marginally inadequate.
D. The STA is used to revascularize the MCA territory only.
E. The occipital artery is most commonly used for bypass to the PICA, but it can also be used to revascularize the AICA as well.

✅ The answer is **D**.
- The STA can be used to revascularize the MCA territory, as well as the distal posterior circulation via the superior cerebellar artery or PCA.
- Pedicled scalp artery is used as the donor vessel.

? 152. **Revascularization procedures for complex aneurysms***
Type IV bypass, the FALSE answer is:
A. Is direct intracranial revascularization.
B. Involves an anastomosis between two adjacent cerebral arteries.

C. This type of procedure can involve end-to-end primary reanastomosis after excision of an aneurysm.
D. Examples include PICA-PICA and pericallosal-pericallosal anastomoses.
E. Examples do not include MCA-MCA and PICA-AICA anastomoses.

✅ The answer is **E.**
- Examples include PICA-PICA, pericallosal-pericallosal, MCA-MCA, and PICA-AICA anastomoses.
- This type of procedure can involve end-to-end primary reanastomosis after excision of an aneurysm, side-to-side anastomosis of two adjacent intracranial arteries, or an end-to side anastomosis between two cerebral arteries.
- Pericallosal-to-pericallosal bypass can be used to treat fusiform aneurysms of the proximal pericallosal artery or for giant anterior communicating artery aneurysms that require trapping. This side-to-side anastomosis serves as a new communicating artery.
- A PICA-to-PICA anastomosis can be used when the occipital artery is small or has been damaged during a previous surgical procedure.

❓ **153.** **Revascularization procedures for complex aneurysms***
Bypass, the FALSE answer is:
A. Normal blood flow of the MCA is about 250 mL/min.
B. Blood flow of saphenous vein graft is 70–140 mL/min.
C. Blood flow of radial artery graft is 40 and 70 mL/min.
D. Blood flow of STA graft is 15–30 mL/min.
E. Average diameter of radial artery graft is larger than saphenous vein graft.

✅ The answer is **E.**
- Radial artery graft can be used, which has a smaller diameter (about **3.5** mm) and a flow rate between 40 and 70 mL/min.
- Blood flow through a saphenous vein graft, which averages about **4–5** mm in diameter, is high enough to support the circulation in an entire major arterial territory at a level well above the ischemic threshold.
- Blood flow of saphenous vein graft typically ranges from 70 to 140 mL/min and can exceed 250 mL/min.

❓ **154.** **Revascularization procedures for complex aneurysms***
Bypass, the FALSE answer is:
A. In saphenous vein graft, it is a must to reverse the ends, so that the distal end in the leg will be the intracranial end.

B. The ideal arterial recipient site of MCA is M2 or M3 (free of perforating vessels).
C. STA-MCA bypass includes a craniotomy centered 6 cm above the external auditory meatus (Chater's point), where several large MCA branches emerge from the distal sylvian fissure.
D. The most serious acute complication is early graft occlusion.
E. If there is any doubt about the integrity of the graft, intraoperative angiography should be considered.

✅ The answer is **A**.
- It is also important to pass the saphenous vein so that the end that was proximal in the leg is the end used for the cranial, distal anastomosis (because of the unidirectional valve arrangement).
- The most serious acute complication is early graft occlusion.
- Rate of ischemic complications and graft occlusion typically exceeds 10 %.
- A normal flow signal should be confirmed with intraoperative Doppler assessment.
- Subdural or epidural hematomas (or both) developed postoperatively. Some of these hematomas were small and asymptomatic.

❓ 155. **Complex cerebrovascular lesions***
Multimodality management, the FALSE answer is:
A. Rates of failed coil embolization were found to be as high as 14.5 % because of an inability to place coils into the aneurysmal sac.
B. Coil embolization intraprocedural mortality rate of 2 % with an overall retreatment rate of 17.4 %.
C. Failure to completely occlude an aneurysm by surgical clipping is up to 5.9 % of procedures.
D. Retreatment rates of the target aneurysm after the first year of coil embolization are lower than that for clipping.
E. Rehemorrhage rates of the target aneurysm after the first year of coil embolization are higher than that for clipping.

✅ The answer is **D**.
- Retreatment and rehemorrhage rates of the target aneurysm after coil embolization within the first year were 7.7 % and 3.0 %, respectively.
- Retreatment and rehemorrhage rates of the target aneurysm within the first year after clipping were found to be 1.7 % and 1.3 %, respectively.
- Further classification of these complex surgical cases of inadequately embolized aneurysms was attempted.

- Group A (65 % of cases) allowed direct surgical clipping.
- Group B (23 % of cases) showed parent vessel narrowing after clip application, which required extraction of coils from the fundus and reconstruction of the neck by clip or suture.
- Group C (12 % of cases) consisted of emergency coil removal after embolization procedures.

? 156. Traumatic intracranial aneurysms (TICA)
The FALSE answer is:
   A. Despite the common occurrence of head trauma, **TICA** are rare entities that represent less than 1 % of all intracranial aneurysms.
   B. 20 % of TICA are multiple.
   C. TICA occur relatively frequently in children.
   D. All TICA have a propensity to bleed at the time of initial trauma.
   E. The anterior circulation is most often affected, with peripheral branches of the MCA being the most frequent site, followed by pericallosal vessels.

✔ The answer is D.
- ICA have a propensity to bleed weeks after the initial trauma.
- Each individual aneurysm may regress, enlarge, or form in delayed fashion.
- In aneurysms involving the peripheral vascular tree, there is delayed neurological deterioration, usually within 3 weeks of the injury.

? 157. TICA
The FALSE answer is:
   A. The term pseudoaneurysm is often used to describe aneurysms related to trauma.
   B. Pseudoaneurysms, which form the majority of TICA, are essentially contained hematomas with disruption of all three layers of the vessel wall.
   C. True aneurysm and a false one are always possible to distinguish them on angiography.
   D. Distinction between a true aneurysm and a false one requires histologic analysis.
   E. TICA occur distally in the vascular tree, and this peripheral location reflects the underlying mechanism of injury.

✅ The answer is **C**.
- True aneurysm and a false one are not always possible to distinguish them on angiography.

❓ **158. TICA**

MECHANISM, the FALSE answer is:

A. The relative incidence of TICA varies according to etiology.
B. TICA may be the result of either penetrating or nonpenetrating trauma.
C. Aneurysm formation being much less likely after closed head injury than after penetrating trauma.
D. Aneurysm formation being less likely after low-velocity than after high-velocity penetrating injuries.
E. TICA have been reported to occur iatrogenically, such as after transsphenoidal surgery and endoscopic third ventriculostomy.

✅ The answer is **D**.
- Aneurysm formation being much more likely after low-velocity penetrating injuries (as knives, screwdrivers) than after high-velocity penetrating injuries caused by missiles.
- The relative incidence of TICA varies according to etiology: blunt trauma in 70 %, penetrating injuries in 20 %, and iatrogenic in about 10 %.
- In addition to their occurrence after traditional trauma, TICA have been reported to occur iatrogenically, such as after transsphenoidal surgery, sinus surgery, ventricular taps, stereotactic brain biopsy, and endoscopic third ventriculostomy.

❓ **159. TICA**

MECHANISM, the FALSE answer is:

A. TICA are 14 times more likely with shrapnel injuries than with bullet injuries, which are of higher velocity.
B. The incidence of aneurysm formation after stab wound type of injury may be as high as 10–12 %.
C. With respect to missile injuries, aneurysm formation in 0.1–8 % of patients sustaining this type of injury.
D. The MCA are most at risk when fractures involve the skull base.
E. Penetrating missile injuries usually affect the supratentorial vessels.

✅ The answer is **D**.
- The petrous and cavernous portions of the ICA are most at risk when fractures involve the skull base.

❓ **160. TICA**
MECHANISM, the FALSE answer is:
A. Severe and life-threatening epistaxis can be the initial event in MCA injury.
B. Because most TICA are false aneurysms, ICH is often the reason for this deterioration.
C. Penetrating trauma is often associated with ICH.
D. After missile injuries, concomitant ICH is found in up to 80 % of patients.
E. In low-velocity penetrating injuries, 50 % of patients had an ICH.

✅ The answer is **A**.
- In patients with aneurysms involving the infraclinoid CA, severe and life-threatening epistaxis can be the initial event if the arterial injury communicates with a sphenoidal sinus fracture.

❓ **161. TICA**
MECHANISM, the FALSE answer is:
A. Cerebral angiography is the "gold standard" and should be performed in all cases of penetrating trauma.
B. Angiography is particularly important in patients with orbitopterional injuries, penetrating fragments, and SAH, ICH, or SDH.
C. In penetrating trauma, traumatic aneurysms may be visualized on angiography as early as 2 h after the injury.
D. In penetrating trauma, the majority of aneurysms are angiographically apparent in the first day.
E. Once a traumatic aneurysm has been diagnosed, therapy should be instituted.

✅ The answer is **D**.
- In penetrating trauma, the majority of aneurysms are angiographically apparent in 2–3 weeks.

? **162.** **TICA**
MANAGEMENT, the FALSE answer is:
A. Surgery is still the mainstay of treatment.
B. Endovascular therapy is becoming an important option, particularly those involving the skull base.
C. TICA may be amenable to either resection or bypass and wrapping.
D. The outcome is related more to the aneurysm itself than to the primary injury.
E. TICA have a mortality rate of 30 %.

✓ The answer is **D**.
- The outcome is related more to the primary injury than to the aneurysm itself.
- Endovascular therapy has not been a mainstay of treatment of TICA in the peripheral vascular tree because of the high incidence of false aneurysms and the risk for rupture.

? **163.** **ACP (anterior clinoid process) drilling during approaches for various intracranial aneurysm**
The FALSE answer is:
A. Anatomically ACP, formed by the medial extension of the lesser wing of the sphenoid bone, provides a bony roof to the superior orbital fissure (SOF) and the anterior cavernous sinus.
B. The optic strut extends from the inferomedial surface of the ACP to the body of the sphenoid bone, separating the optic canal from the SOF.
C. The ACP is thus connected to the skull at two main points of bony fixation: the medial aspect of the lesser sphenoid wing and the optic strut.
D. The ACP and optic strut define and obstruct access to the anterior and lateral borders of the ascending ICA.
E. The superomedial portion of the ACP is connected to the planum sphenoidale by the roof of the optic canal, the most posterior portion of which is formed by a dural fold called the falciform ligament.

✓ The answer is **C**.
- The ACP is thus connected to the skull at **three** main points of bony fixation: the medial aspect of the lesser sphenoid wing, the optic strut, and the roof of the optic canal.

164. **ACP drilling* during skull base approaches for various intracranial aneurysms**
The FALSE answer is:

A. The direction of the drilling is from lateral to medial.
B. The optic strut is drilled and the clinoid process freed from its bony fixation points.
C. During ACP drilling, orbitomeningeal artery bleeding indicates proximity to the SOF.
D. Venous bleeding from the lateral cavernous sinus wall is common during the procedure and generally responds to tamponade and pressures them by Surgicel or Gelfoam.
E. Thermal injury can occur during drilling of the ACP and is prevented by generous irrigation to dissipate the heat or by using the newer ultrasonic bone aspirators.

✔ The answer is **A**.
- The direction of the drilling is from medial to lateral (from the optic nerve toward the superior orbital fissure).
- The orbitomeningeal artery can be coagulated and divided.
- Irrigation is not only necessary to prevent thermal injury but also to clear bone dust while drilling.

165. **ACP drilling* during skull base approaches for various intracranial aneurysm**
The FALSE answer is:

A. Anterior clinoidectomy has great value in the surgical exposure and treatment for most paraclinoid aneurysms.
B. ACP removal can be performed through an extradural (ED) or intradural (ID) approach determined primarily by the relationship between the aneurysm and ACP.
C. The ID ACP resection is preferable in most instances because it allows the surgeon to see the optic nerve and aneurysm during the entire dissection.
D. ID ACP removal is preferred for large, complex, or ruptured aneurysms.
E. ED ACP removal is not feasible for ophthalmic segment aneurysms.

✔ The answer is **E**.
- ED ACP removal is feasible for most ophthalmic segment aneurysms.

166. **ACP drilling* during skull base approaches for various intracranial aneurysm**
The FALSE answer is:
A. ED ACP: before the dura is opened, the posterior half of the roof and lateral wall of the orbit and the sphenoid ridge over the SOF are removed to define the orbital portion of the optic nerve.
B. ED ACP: before the dura is opened, the ACP is internally cavitated using a small (3 mm) diamond drill, and the remaining thin remnants are removed with small rongeurs and curettes.
C. ID ACP: the roof and lateral wall of the orbit and the sphenoid ridge are removed extradurally.
D. ID ACP: once the dura is opened, the sylvian fissure is split widely from lateral to medial to expose the ICA and the ACP.
E. All of the above are true.

The answer is **E**.

167. **ACP drilling* during skull base approaches for various intracranial aneurysm**
The FALSE answer is:
A. ID ACP: a dural incision is then made along the lesser sphenoid wing extending from the tip of the ACP laterally beyond the edge of the prior ridge resection.
B. ID ACP: a second dural incision made perpendicular to the first near the clinoid tip extends to and includes sectioning of the falciform ligament.
C. ID ACP: the ACP and optic canal roof and lateral wall then are thinned with a small diamond bur, and the remaining bone is removed with small rongeurs.
D. ID ACP: the ACP is exposed by retracting the dural leaflets and then is removed in a similar fashion as the extradural removal, but with better visualization of the optic apparatus and the aneurysm.
E. ID ACP: finally, the optic strut is drilled to expose the petrous part of ICA.

The answer is **E**.
 − ID ACP: finally, the optic strut is drilled to expose the anterior border of the clinoidal segment of the ICA.

168. ACP drilling* during skull base approaches for various intracranial aneurysm
The FALSE answer is:

A. CSF rhinorrhea can also occur when the optic strut is pneumatized with a fingerlike projection from the sphenoid sinus (optico-carotid recess) that is opened during strut removal.

B. This anatomy, occurring in 4–13 % of patients, results in a communication between the subarachnoid space and the sphenoid sinus.

C. Adequate removal of the optic strut should be compromised if there is any concern for postoperative CSF rhinorrhea.

D. This CSF rhinorrhea can be repaired with the "yo-yo" technique.

E. Application of this technique does not require preoperative preparations, only the intraoperative recognition of a pneumatized strut.

The answer is **C.**

– Adequate removal of the optic strut and thorough dissection of the distal dural ring is critical to clipping OphA aneurysms and should not be compromised by concern for postoperative CSF rhinorrhea.

– The yo-yo technique, named because sutured muscle resembles a yo-yo in both form and motion, reverses the usual direction of muscle packing, pulling the muscle from the sphenoid sinus into the optic strut. Pulling a plug into the funnel-shaped anatomy is more effective mechanically than pushing a plug out of a funnel.

– Removal of the anterior clinoid process may cause postoperative CSF leak, especially when the anterior clinoid is well pneumatized and communicates with the ethmoidal sinuses. Bone wax should be applied to the open sinuses to obliterate any potential opening in them.

169. Fusiform aneurysm (FA)
DEFINITION, the FALSE answer is:

A. Fusiform aneurysms are dilated, tortuous, and elongated arterial segments.

B. Fusiform aneurysms are characterized by circumferential involvement of the parent artery.

C. Fusiform aneurysms are also characterized by a well-defined neck.

D. The spectrum of fusiform aneurysms may arise from congenital, acquired, or iatrogenic defects in the vessel wall.

E. Distinct subgroups of fusiform aneurysms are serpentine aneurysms, large and partially thrombosed tortuous aneurysms with a central parent channel, eccentrically located within the intraluminal clot.

✓ The answer is **C.**
- Fusiform aneurysms are characterized by circumferential involvement of the parent artery, the absence of a defined neck, and a longish course.
- The spectrum of fusiform aneurysms may arise from congenital, acquired, or iatrogenic defects in the vessel wall, with or without atherosclerosis, and hypertension, or may develop after intimal tear from dissection.
- Distinct subgroups of fusiform aneurysms are serpentine aneurysms, large and partially thrombosed tortuous aneurysms with a central parent channel, eccentrically located within the intraluminal clot. This channel is not endothelialized and does not contain elastic lamina or media. The etiology of serpentine aneurysms is still totally unclear.
- They may develop from a degenerative form of atherosclerosis, infection, or may be congenital. They occur most commonly in the internal carotid artery, the middle cerebral artery, and posterior cerebral artery. Typically, they present with symptoms of mass effect. Subarachnoid or intracerebral hemorrhage is rare.

? 170. **Fusiform aneurysm (FA)**
DEFINITION, the FALSE answer is:
A. FA is defined as a circumferential arterial dilatation resulting from pathological involvement of the entire artery.
B. Aneurysms exhibit a spindle shape when viewed externally.
C. There is a female predominance.
D. There is a male predominance.
E. The mean age of patients is 45 years.

✓ The answer is **C.**
- The male/female ratio is 1.4:1. This contrasts with that of patients with saccular aneurysms.

? 171. **Fusiform aneurysm (FA)**
The FALSE answer is:
A. Dissection has been proposed as the main underlying cause of FAs.
B. Dissecting FA most commonly involves the posterior circulation, especially vertebral and basilar arteries.

C. Dissecting FA most frequently occurs in the distal vertebral artery, basilar artery, P1 segment of the PCA, and the supraclinoid ICA.

D. About 75 % of spontaneous FAs are seen in the anterior circulation and the rest in the posterior circulation.

E. The vertebral artery is the most common site for spontaneous FAs.

✅ The answer is **E**.
- The MCA is the most common site for spontaneous FAs (75 %).

❓ **172. Fusiform aneurysm (FA)**
PRESENTATION, the FALSE answer is:
A. Hemorrhage is the most common presentation in patients with small lesions with focal dilatation.

B. Hemorrhage is the most common presentation of patients with stenosis or occluded vessels.

C. FA can be incidental or asymptomatic, discovered during work-up for unrelated symptoms.

D. Presenting symptoms such as cranial neuropathy, brain stem compression, and cerebral ischemia are mainly due to mass effect and distal embolization.

E. FA of the vertebral artery can present with hemifacial spasm due to mass effect.

✅ The answer is **B**.
- Ischemic symptoms are the most common presentation of patients with stenosis or occluded vessels.

❓ **173. Fusiform aneurysm (FA)**
MANAGEMENT, the FALSE answer is:
A. Most small and some large focal dilatations, especially asymptomatic, should be treated conservatively.

B. Patients with stenotic or occlusive lesions presenting with acute ischemic symptoms should be treated conservatively.

C. Conservative treatment is recommended in patients with dissecting aneurysms without neurological deterioration or recurrent SAH.

D. The appearance of symptoms does not signify the need for intervention.

E. FA is usually not suitable for endovascular obliteration because they do not have a circumscribed neck.

✅ The answer is **D**.
- The appearance of symptoms **requires aggressive intervention.**
- Aggressive surgical treatment is recommended for FAs which are not caused by dissection (possible progression).
- Proximal occlusion or trapping with or without resection combined with end-to-end anastomosis or external carotid-internal carotid (EC-IC) bypass, but there is no consensus on this issue.
- In selected cases, endovascular parent vessel occlusion may be a therapeutic option, particularly if mass effect is the leading symptom. The aneurysm may subsequently shrink in size or completely resolve.

Arteriovenous Malformations

This book contains some difficult questions marked with " * " sign.

© Springer International Publishing AG 2017
S.S. Hoz, *Vascular Neurosurgery*, DOI 10.1007/978-3-319-49187-5_2

1. The most common intracerebral vascular malformations
The TRUE answer is:
A. AVMs
B. Cavernous malformation
C. Venous angioma
D. Capillary telangiectasia
E. Aneurysm

✔ The answer is **C.**
- DVA or venous angiomas are the most common intracerebral vascular malformation in general and also in autopsy.

2. AVMs
Definition, the FALSE answer is:
A. True AVMs are abnormalities of the intracranial vessels in which the arterial and venous systems are connected without an intervening capillary bed.
B. Mainly congenital lesions which develop during the late somite stage, between the fourth week and the eighth week of embryonic life.
C. The AVMs are the most common clinically (or surgically) significant vascular malformation.
D. They are high-flow, high-pressure lesions.
E. Never contains parenchymal tissue within the nidus.

✔ The answer is **E.**
- There may be parenchymal element within the nidus but if present tend to be gliotic, hemosiderin stained, and nonfunctional.
- **AVMs are mainly congenital in origin but the presentation is usually at adult life.**
- **AVMs are high flow and high pressure especially in adult.**

3. AVMs
Location, the FALSE answer is:
A. Supratentorial in 85 % and infratentorial in 15 %.
B. Parietal area is the most common region involved in supratentorial lesions.
C. Hemispheric AVMs are located in the MCA, PCA, and ACA territories in declining frequencies.
D. The location of the base in most AVMs is periventricular.
E. There is no significant hemispheric preference.

✅ The answer is **D**.
- The location of the **apex** in most AVMs is periventricular because small arteries from the ependymal surface feed the AVM. The AVM base usually faces the cortex.
- Also the parietal area is the most common location of AVM to give rise to seizures followed by insula, frontal, and temporal lobes.
- Superficial is slightly more than deep AVMs.
- The eloquent location is slightly more than non-eloquent.

❓ 4. AVMs
Pathology, the FALSE answer is:
A. Classic morphologic features are feeding arteries, draining veins, and a dysplastic vascular nidus composed of a tangle of abnormal vessels.
B. The AVMs fed predominantly by the trans-cerebral vessels.
C. AVMs classically assume the shape of a cone (wedge), based on the cortical surface with its apex often reaching the ventricular wall.
D. Most AVMs demonstrate a gliotic core associated with the nidus.
E. Most AVMs demonstrate a gliotic wall around the malformation forming a "true capsule" which helps in surgical dissection.

✅ The answer is **E**.
- Most AVMs demonstrate a gliotic core associated with the nidus and a gliotic wall around the malformation forming a "false capsule" which helps in surgical dissection.
- A type of proliferative or diffuse AVM without a focal nidus is often seen in pediatric patients.

❓ 5. AVMs
Pathology, the FALSE answer is:
A. Dilation and tortuosity of feeding arteries.
B. Smooth muscle hyperplasia associated with fibroblasts and connective tissue elements known as fibromuscular cushions.
C. Vascular or interstitial calcification of the vessel in an AVM is never occurring.
D. Thickening of the vein due to collagenous tissue is usually noted and thrombosis may be found.
E. Arteries and arterialized veins may be difficult to distinguish from one another.

✅ The answer is **C**.
- Vascular or interstitial calcification of vessel in an AVM is common to occur.

? 6. AVMs

Natural history, the FALSE answer is:

A. The average age of patients diagnosed with AVMs is around 30 years.
B. Large AVMs tend to present more often as hemorrhages than do small ones.
C. The annual rebleed rate is 2–4 %.
D. The annual mortality rate is 1 %.
E. Spontaneous closure may occur.

✓ The answer is B.

- Small AVMs tend to present more often as hemorrhages than do large ones.
- The incidence of first bleed for unruptured AVM or the annual rebleed rate or lifelong risk of bleeding per year is 2–4 %, while the risk of rebleed from an AVM in the first year is as high as 5–15 %.
- Because of the higher pressures in the feeding artery, it was postulated that larger AVMs presented as seizure more often simply because their size made them more likely to involve the cortex.
- The combined annual morbidity plus mortality from AVMs is approximately 2 %, the annual mortality rate is 1 %, the mortality at each bleed is 10 %, and the morbidity for each bleed is 30 to 50 %.
- About statement E, the exact mechanisms involved in spontaneous AVM regression are uncertain but the most common is compression of the lesion (leading to acute intravascular thrombosis) from intracranial hemorrhage.
- Several factors appear to be associated with spontaneous occlusion of cerebral AVM: single draining vein (84 % of cases of spontaneous occlusion), solitary arterial feeder (30 %), and small size of the nidus (<3 cm in 50 %).

? 7. AVMs

Clinical features, the FALSE answer is:

A. 15 % of AVMs have no symptoms.
B. The most common presentation of AVM is ICH then seizures and less likely headache, stroke, or neurological deficit.
C. Common cause of SAH.
D. The older the patient at diagnosis, the higher the risk of developing convulsions.
E. The factor that is significantly different in pediatric age group is the initial mode of presentation, with bleeding outnumbering other symptoms in children.

✔ The answer is **D**.

- The younger the patient at diagnosis, the higher the risk of developing convulsions.
- The factor that is significantly different between the pediatric and adult age groups is the initial mode of presentation, with bleed (90 %) outnumbering other symptoms in children.

❓ 8. **AVMs**

Factors that increase the risk of bleeding of AVMs, the FALSE answer is:
A. High feeding artery pressure
B. Aneurysm or deep venous drainage
C. Increasing age or pediatric patients or pregnancy or history of hypertension
D. Arterial border zone location of brain AVMs
E. Residual nidus after surgery or Spetzler-Martin grade IV or V AVMs.

✔ The answer is **D**.

- Arterial border zone location of brain AVMs is an independent determinant of lower risk of incident AVMs hemorrhage.

❓ 9. **AVMs**

Anatomic factors that increase the risk of bleeding of AVMs, the FALSE answer is:
A. Aneurysm (feeding artery and intranidal aneurysms)
B. Nidus (diffuse morphology and small-size AVM)
C. Venous recruitment
D. Location (deep locations, periventricular, intraventricular space, and infratentorial)
E. Impaired venous drainage

✔ The answer is **C**.

Factors that increase the risk of bleeding of AVMs:
- Anatomic factors:
  1. Aneurysm (feeding artery and intranidal aneurysms)
  2. Nidus (diffuse morphology)
  3. Location (deep locations, periventricular, intraventricular space, and infratentorial)
  4. Impaired venous drainage: deep venous drainage, venous stenosis, single draining vein, and venous reflux into a sinus or a deep vein
  5. Small-size AVM

- Hemodynamic factors: high feeding artery pressure
- Patient factors: increasing age, pediatric patients, pregnancy, history of hypertension
- Others: residual nidus after surgery, Hispanic race/ethnicity, Spetzler-Martin grade IV or V AVMs

Factors that decrease the risk of bleeding of AVMs:
1. Arterial stenosis
2. Arterial angioectasia
3. Arterial border zone location of brain AVMs
4. Venous recruitment

The risk of AVM bleeding (at least once) over one's lifetime:
- Lifetime risk (%) = 105 – the patient's age in years
- (Assuming approximately a 2 to 4 %/year bleed rate)

❓ 10. AVMs AND PREGNANCY
   The FALSE answer is:
   A. Hemorrhage secondary to AVM rupture remains a major cause of non-obstetric morbidity and mortality in pregnant women.
   B. Up to 50 % of pregnant women presenting with intracranial hemorrhage have ruptured AVMs.
   C. The course of AVM rupture may actually be more aggressive in pregnant patients when compared to nongravid women.
   D. If a pregnant patient presents with a hemorrhage from an AVM, the risk of rebleed during the same pregnancy can be up to 27 %.
   E. The rupture of AVMs in pregnant women may occur frequently in the first trimester.

✅ The answer is **E.**
   - There is also evidence that rupture of AVMs in pregnant women may occur frequently between week 20 of gestation and 6 weeks postpartum (more in third trimester) and may be attributable to hemodynamic, hormonal, and coagulation changes that occur during this time.
   - If a pregnant patient presents with a hemorrhage from an AVM, the risk of rebleed during the same pregnancy can be up to 27 %.

❓ 11. AVMs and pregnancy
   The FALSE answer is:
   A. Maternal mortality exceeded fetal mortality.
   B. The supine position is poorly tolerated during pregnancy because of vascular congestion.

C. Mannitol and furosemide should not be administered judiciously during craniotomy in pregnant women.
D. There is no role for radiosurgery in the treatment of pregnant women, whether the AVM is ruptured or unruptured.
E. The risk to the fetus and the slow rate of occlusion make radiosurgery not a viable option during pregnancy.

✅ The answer is **C**.
— Mannitol and furosemide should be administered judiciously during craniotomy in pregnant women because diuresis may create significant fluid shifts for the fetus that are potentially detrimental.

❓ 12. **AVM-associated aneurysms**
Types, the FALSE answer is:
A. Remote: unrelated to flow vessels.
B. Proximal: arising at the circle of Willis origin of a vessel supplying the AVM.
C. Pedicular: arising from the midcourse of a feeding pedicle.
D. Intranidal: arising from within the nidus itself.
E. Flow-unrelated are more common than flow-related aneurysms.

✅ The answer is **E**.
— The proximal, pedicular, and intranidal types can be classified as "flow-related" aneurysms. Flow related is 85 %; flow unrelated is 15 %.

❓ 13. **AVM-associated aneurysms**
The FALSE answer is:
A. About 9.9 % of AVMs are associated with an aneurysm.
B. 75 % of these aneurysms are located on major feeding artery of AVMs.
C. More aneurysms appear to occur, however, in association with larger AVMs.
D. The frequency of associated aneurysms with AVMs decreased with patient age.
E. The increased flow is believed to influence the incidence of the association of AVMs and aneurysms.

✅ The answer is **D**.
— The frequency of associated aneurysms with AVMs increased with patient age.
— About 9.9 % (7–20 %) of AVMs are associated with an aneurysm.

- Gender appears to have no influence on the incidence.
- Patient age, size of the AVM, and increased flow are believed to influence the incidence of the association of AVMs and aneurysms.

? 14. AVM-associated aneurysms
The FALSE answer is:
   A. Multiple aneurysms appear to occur more frequently when an AVM is present.
   B. 66 % of the aneurysms regress after AVM removal.
   C. Aneurysms close to the nidus have a higher rate of spontaneous regression after AVM resection than proximal ones.
   D. In tandem AVM and aneurysm, the symptomatic one is usually treated first.
   E. When feasible, both tandem AVM and aneurysm may be treated at same operation.

✓ The answer is **C.**
- Aneurysms close to the nidus (distal flow related) have a lower rate of spontaneous regression after AVM resection than proximal ones.
- When an aneurysm reaches the clinical threshold for treatment, the aneurysm should be treated first because resection of the AVM may increase the risk of rupture of the aneurysm by increasing distal resistance and transmural gradient. Conversely, at the time of the aneurysm repair, care must be taken with fluid and blood pressure management, as AVM rupture has been reported after aneurysm surgery.
- Symptomatic intranidal aneurysms may be addressed by selective embolization of the portion of the nidus containing the aneurysm before surgery or radiosurgery of the entire AVM or in untreatable AVMs where securing the intranidal aneurysm may lower the natural history risk of hemorrhage of AVM.

? 15. AVMs vs. aneurysms (comparison)
The FALSE answer is:
   A. The average age of patients diagnosed with AVMs is around 33 years, which is 10 years younger than that of aneurysms.
   B. Hemorrhage in AVMs is 50 % compared to 90 % for aneurysms.
   C. Cerebral AVMs produce more SAH than aneurysms.
   D. Of patients with an aneurysm, roughly 1 % also harbors an intracranial AVM.
   E. Of patients with an AVM, 10 % have one or more intracranial aneurysms.

✅ The answer is **C**.
- Cerebral AVMs second to aneurysms among the intracranial vascular lesions that produce SAH with relative incidence (aneurysm/AVM is 10:1 to 4:1).
- The risk of aneurysm re-rupture is higher in the acute setting, and the risk of morbidity and death from an aneurysmal subarachnoid hemorrhage is higher compared to an AVM.

❓ 16. **AVMs**
   In pediatrics, the FALSE answer is:
   A. Children form 15–33 % of all AVM patients.
   B. The second most common cause of spontaneous ICH in children is AVM rupture.
   C. Hemorrhage is by far the most common initial manifestation of the lesion.
   D. AVMs in pediatric patients tend to be smaller and located superficially.
   E. AVMs were more common in male pediatric patients.

✅ The answer is **B**.
- The most common cause of spontaneous ICH in children is AVM rupture.
- Hemorrhage is by far the most common initial manifestation of the lesion (50–90 %), followed by seizures (8–25 %) and congestive heart failure (18 %).
- Hemorrhage and seizures occur more frequently in children older than 2 years.
- Even though 68 % of pediatric patients with AVMs suffered hemorrhage, only 6 % had deep venous drainage.
- AVMs can grow in size, and this is usually most prominent in the pediatric age group.

❓ 17. **AVMs**
   In pediatrics, the FALSE answer is:
   A. The mortality associated with AVM hemorrhage in children is high.
   B. The higher mortality in pediatric series may relate to the posterior fossa AVMs.
   C. Children are less likely than adults to improve after intracerebral hemorrhage caused by AVM rupture.
   D. Neonates with congestive heart failure usually have residual shunting after treatment.
   E. Neonates with congestive heart failure have a very poor prognosis.

✅ The answer is **C**.
- Despite high mortality rates, children are more likely than adults to improve after intracerebral hemorrhage caused by AVM rupture.

❓ **18. AVM-associated syndromes**
The FALSE answer is:
A. Osler-Weber-Rendu syndrome
B. Tuberous sclerosis
C. Sturge-Weber syndrome
D. Klippel-Trenaunay syndrome
E. AD polycystic kidney disease

✅ The answer is **B**.
- Tuberous sclerosis is not a known associated syndrome with AVMs.
- Other associated syndromes include: Wyburn-Mason syndrome, Bannayan syndrome, and Parks-Weber syndrome.

❓ **19. AVMs**
Radiology, the FALSE answer is:
A. Plain CT scan usually does not show "parenchymatous calcifications."
B. Plain CT scan may show "nidus sparing sign."
C. Plain CT scan may show "bag of worms."
D. MRI may show "honeycomb" of flow voids.
E. The angiographic hallmark of AVMs is the "early draining vein."

✅ The answer is **A**.
- Plain CT scan may show "parenchymatous calcifications" in majority of AVMs.

❓ **20. AVMs**
Radiology, the FALSE answer is:
A. MR sequence that best shows hemosiderin ring is gradient echo MRI.
B. MRA play an important role in the follow-up of AVMs following radio-surgical ablation.
C. The presence of significant edema around the lesion may indicate an AVM rather than a tumor that has bled.
D. The presence of hemosiderin ring of low density surrounding the lesion suggests AVM over tumor.
E. Digital subtraction angiography is considered the "gold standard" in the imaging of AVMs.

✔ The answer is **C**.
— The presence of significant edema around the lesion may indicate a tumor rather than an AVM that has bled.
— MRA plays an important role in the follow-up of AVMs following radio-surgical ablation, resulting in a reduction in the number of required post-therapeutic catheter angiograms.

❓ 21. **AVMs**
Radiology, the FALSE answer is:
A. In ruptured AVM, CT in the acute phase shows high specificity for hemorrhage.
B. In ruptured AVM, the next step after the diagnosis of the hemorrhage is selective angiography.
C. In ruptured AVM, contrast-enhanced CT and CT angiography are very essential.
D. In unruptured AVM, CT is not indicated; the first step is MRI and MRA to obtain all the information needed to make a therapeutic decision.
E. In unruptured AVM, if the therapeutic decision is not clear after MRI and MRA, angiography is performed to make a decision.

✔ The answer is **C**.
— In ruptured AVM, contrast-enhanced CT scan and CT angiography are not useful.
— In ruptured AVM, after the acute phase of bleeding, the therapeutic approach to the AVM will be defined on the basis of anatomic data provided by MRI and selective angiography.

❓ 22. **AVMs*, grading, 45-year-old male presented to the emergency room with right 5 cm frontopolar AVM.**
On angiography, this AVM is noted to have superficial drainage.
How would one best grade this AVM according to Spetzler-Martin grading?
A. 1
B. 2
C. 3
D. 4
E. 5

✔ The answer is **B**.

Spetzler-Martin grading system for AVM	
Feature	**Points assigned**
Size of AVM	
Small (< 3 cm)	1
Medium (3–6 cm)	2
Large (> 6 cm)	3
Eloquence of adjacent brain	
Non-eloquent	0
Eloquent	1
Pattern of venous drainage	
Superficial only	0
Deep	1

Surgical outcome predicted by Spetzler-Martin grading system			
S-M grade	**No deficits (%)**	**Minor deficits (%)**	**Major deficits (%)**
1	100	0	0
2	95	5	0
3	84	12	4
4	73	20	7
5	69	19	12

Three-tier classification of cerebral AVM		
Class	**S-M grade**	**Management**
A	I, II	Surgical resection
B	III	Multimodality treatment
C	IV, V	No treatment

Exceptions for the treatment of class C AVMs include recurrent hemorrhages, progressive neurological deficits, steal-related symptoms, and AVM-related aneurysms

❓ 23. *About the case in MCQ no. 22, if you know that this AVM drains via several stenotic veins, how would one best grade this AVM?
   A. Spetzler-Martin grade 2A
   B. Spetzler-Martin grade 2B
   C. Spetzler-Martin grade 3A
   D. Spetzler-Martin grade 3B
   E. Spetzler-Martin grade 5A

✔️ The answer is **A**.
   ▬ The fact that it has stenotic venous drainage gives it a subclassification of 2A.

❓ 24. *About the case in MCQ no. 22, what is the class of this AVM according to Spetzler-Ponce classification (AVM grading and treatment)?
   A. A
   B. B
   C. C
   D. D
   E. E

✔️ The answer is **A**.
   Spetzler-Ponce classification (AVM grading and treatment) (2010):
   ▬ **Class A**
      ▬ Spetzler-Martin score 1 or 2.
      ▬ Microsurgical resection is preferred treatment.
      ▬ 8 % chance on postoperative deficit (95 % CI = 6–10).
   ▬ **Class B**
      ▬ Spetzler-Martin score 3
      ▬ Multimodality treatment
      ▬ 18 % chance on postoperative deficit (95 % CI = 15–22)
   ▬ **Class C**
      ▬ Spetzler-Martin score 4–5
      ▬ No treatment, with exception of recurrent hemorrhages, progressive neurological deficits, steal-related symptoms, and AVM-related aneurysms
      ▬ 32 % chance on postoperative deficit (95 % CI = 27–38)

❓ 25. *About the case in MCQ no. 22, if you know that this AVM is ruptured and on angiography is compact in architecture, what is the supplemental (i.e., Lawton-Young) grade of the patient's AVM?
   A. 1
   B. 2
   C. 3
   D. 4
   E. 5

✅ The answer is **C**.

Supplemental (i.e., Lawton-Young) grading system for AVM	
Feature	**Points assigned**
Age	
<20 years	1
20–40 years	2
>40 years	3
Unruptured presentation	
No	0
Yes	1
Diffuse	
No	0
Yes	1

❓ 26. *About the case in MCQ no. 22, what is the supplemented Spetzler-Martin grade?
  A. 5
  B. 6
  C. 7
  D. 8
  E. 9

✅ The answer is **A**.

❓ 27. *What is the cutoff score for operability of AVMs in the supplemented Spetzler-Martin grading system?
  A. 2
  B. 4
  C. 6
  D. 8
  E. 10

✅ The answer is **C**.

? 28. AVMs

Treatment, the FALSE answer is:

A. Stereotactic radiosurgery may take 1 to 3 years to work during which the patient is still at risk of bleeding from the AVM.

B. Stereotactic radiosurgery should be considered for small AVMs in eloquent cortex.

C. Embolization of AVM prior to stereotactic radiosurgery increases obliteration rate.

D. Common reasons for incomplete obliteration of the nidus are targeting errors and low radiation dose.

E. If bleeding does occur after angiographically documented AVM obliteration, the clinical sequelae are generally minimal.

The answer is C.

- Embolization of AVM prior to stereotactic radiosurgery reduces obliteration rate.

- Common reasons for incomplete obliteration of the nidus are targeting errors, recanalization of a portion of the AVM that was previously embolized, expansion of the nidus after hemorrhage, and low radiation dose.

- If bleeding does occur after angiographically documented AVM obliteration, the clinical sequelae are generally minimal, with the hemorrhages behaving more like bleeding from CMs than AVMs.

? 29. AVMs

Treatment, the FALSE answer is:

A. Surgical resection is the preferred treatment after a recent ICH if the nidus is accessible.

B. Surgery eliminates the risk of bleeding almost immediately.

C. Propranolol used for 3 days prior to AVM resection can minimize the incidence of postop normal perfusion pressure breakthrough.

D. Around 80 % of patients experience an improvement in seizure management after surgery.

E. New neurological deficits account for nearly 10 % of the complications of surgery.

The answer is E.

- New neurological deficits account for nearly 80 % of the complications of surgery.

Dural Arteriovenous Fistula and Carotid-Cavernous Fistula

This book contains some difficult questions marked with " * " sign.

© Springer International Publishing AG 2017
S.S. Hoz, *Vascular Neurosurgery*, DOI 10.1007/978-3-319-49187-5_3

3.1   Dural Arteriovenous Fistula

? 1.   DAVFs (dural arteriovenous fistula (dural AVMs))
   General, the FALSE answer is:
   A.   DAVFs are acquired vascular malformations that are distinct from parenchymal AVMs.
   B.   DAVFs comprise 10–15 % of all intracranial AVMs.
   C.   Patients are typically seen initially between the ages of 40 and 60.
   D.   DAVFs occur more common in females.
   E.   DAVFs are usually multiple.

✓ The answer is **E.**
   − DAVFs are usually solitary, but multiplicity has been reported in about 8 % of cases.
   − DAVFs occur more common in females (61–66 %).

? 2.   DAVFs
   General, the FALSE answer is:
   A.   The most frequent sites for DAVFs are the transverse and sigmoid sinus, anterior cranial base, and tentorium.
   B.   The transverse/sigmoid location is the most common site.
   C.   Carotid-cavernous and transverse/sigmoid DAVFs are more common in women.
   D.   Anterior fossa and tentorial DAVFs are more common in men.
   E.   Usually found adjacent to dural venous sinuses and more in right side.

✓ The answer is **E.**
   − Usually found adjacent to dural venous sinuses. Most common transverse sinus (63 %) and more in left side (usually at the transverse and sigmoid junction).
   − The transverse/sigmoid location is the most common and represents more than 50 % of DAVFs.

? 3.   DAVFs
   Pathology, the FALSE answer is:
   A.   DAVFs consist of a nidus of arteriovenous shunting within the leaflets of the dura mater, in proximity or continuity to a major dural venous sinus or cortical vein.
   B.   These fistulas are frequently congenital.

   C. Grossly, the dural arteries are thickened and the veins dilated in an abnormal vascular network within the wall of a venous sinus.

   D. Fistulas may be high or low flow.

   E. Fistulas may have unilateral or bilateral supply.

✅ The answer is **B**.

   — These fistulas are frequently idiopathic but can be acquired causes like venous thrombosis, trauma, tumor, cranial surgery, sinus infection or meningitis, or association with meningiomas.

   — Demyelination may be seen around leptomeningeal veins as a result of venous hypertension which can lead to leptomeningeal retrograde drainage and predispose these channels to become varicose and potentially rupture.

❓ 4. **DAVFs**

   Natural history, the FALSE answer is:

   A. DAVFs are classified as high or low risk based on the pattern of venous drainage.

   B. DAVFs with retrograde drainage or cortical venous drainage are typically considered to be associated less frequently with ICH.

   C. Untreated DAVFs have an annual hemorrhage rate of 1.6 %.

   D. Persistence of cortical venous reflux in intracranial DAVFs carries an annual risk for neurological deficits of 15 %.

   E. Persistence of cortical venous reflux in intracranial DAVFs carries an annual mortality rate of 10 %.

✅ The answer is **B**.

   — DAVFs with retrograde drainage or cortical venous drainage are typically considered to be associated more frequently with ICH, thus warranting more aggressive treatment.

❓ 5. **DAVFs**

   Natural history (risk factors for hemorrhage), the FALSE answer is:

   A. Cortical venous drainage

   B. Focal neurological deficits

   C. DAVFs located in the anterior fossa

   D. Male sex

   E. Increasing age

✓ The answer is **C.**

- DAVFs located in the posterior fossa are a risk factor for hemorrhage, not the anterior fossa.
- Five risk factors for hemorrhage are cortical venous drainage, focal neurological deficits, DAVFs located in the posterior fossa, male sex, and increasing age.

? 6. **DAVFs**
Clinical features, the FALSE answer is:
A. Patients with DAVFs are frequently asymptomatic.
B. The most common initial symptoms are pulse-synchronous tinnitus and headache.
C. Tinnitus is frequent with carotid-cavernous DAVFs.
D. DAVFs can be accompanied by ICH, seizures, and focal neurological deficits, similar to pial AVMs.
E. Intracranial hemorrhage as the initial symptom is less common.
F. Dural sinus hypertension can produce elevated ICP by impeding cerebral venous drainage.

✓ The answer is **C.**

- Proptosis (especially pulsatile) is frequent with carotid-cavernous DAVFs.
- Pulse-synchronous tinnitus is nearly always exacerbated by a Valsalva maneuver.
- Dural sinus hypertension can produce elevated ICP by impeding cerebral venous drainage and by impairing the function of the arachnoid granulations (which can also lead to hydrocephalus).

? 7. **DAVFs**
Clinical features, the FALSE answer is:
A. Pulsatile tinnitus is the most common initial symptom.
B. Tinnitus occurs because of recruitment of arterial feeders by the DAVF and its close proximity to the middle ear.
C. A bruit can often be auscultated over the cranium.
D. Compression of the carotid artery may result in a reduction in bruit intensity.
E. A change in a bruit (either worsening or disappearance) confirms complete healing.

✅ The answer is **E**.
- Change in a bruit (either worsening or disappearance) should prompts restudy.
- Pulsatile tinnitus is the most common initial symptom and is frequently associated with high-flow fistulas in the transverse sinus/sigmoid location.
- Compression of the carotid artery and jugular vein or occipital artery may result in a reduction in bruit intensity and provide a clue to the diagnosis.

❓ 8. **DAVFs**
Radiology, the FALSE answer is:
A. Findings on CT are often normal.
B. If the fistula drains to cortical veins, contrast-enhanced CT may demonstrate serpiginous enhancement.
C. CT can miss DAVF but not the MRI.
D. MRI can characterize the anatomy and areas of ischemia and chronic hemorrhage.
E. Evidence of dilated cortical veins in MRI may suggest a DAVF with venous hypertension.

✅ The answer is **C**.
- Both MRI and CT can miss DAVF, especially if small or if the DAVF drains into the ipsilateral venous sinus.
- Findings on CT are often normal, although it is the most sensitive in evaluating acute subarachnoid, subdural, or intraparenchymal blood.

❓ 9. **DAVFs**
Radiology, the FALSE answer is:
A. Angiography is the "gold standard" for diagnosis and delineation of the details of the arterial supply and venous drainage.
B. Premature appearance during early arterial phase of a venous structure within or adjacent to dura mater is characteristic.
C. The pattern of venous drainage is the most critical factor.
D. As a rule, lesions with retrograde flow in the cortical veins are high risk for bleeding or intracranial hypertension.
E. Injection includes internal carotid arteries only.

✅ The answer is **E**.
- Injection must include the vertebral and internal and external carotid arteries because DAVF may be overlooked with conventional studies alone.

❓ 10.   **DAVFs**
Borden classification, the FALSE answer is:
- A. Type I fistulas have anterograde drainage into a dural venous sinus or meningeal vein.
- B. Type I fistulas are benign, often asymptomatic or characterized by a cranial bruit.
- C. Type I fistulas have a high rate of spontaneous remission and can be observed.
- D. If conservative treatment is chosen, patients are advised to increase the doses of antiplatelet or anticoagulant agents.
- E. Compression therapy is seldom used currently.

✅ The answer is **D**.
- If conservative treatment is chosen, patients are advised to avoid antiplatelet or anticoagulant agents, if possible, to prevent interference with spontaneous thrombosis of the DAVF.
- Borden type I DAVFs have a high rate of spontaneous remission and can be observed, especially since they may spontaneously thrombose, which has been noted with cavernous sinus DAVFs.
- Compression therapy is seldom used currently, except in patients with Borden type I fistulas as a possible first step before neuroendovascular therapy.
- Compression of the ipsilateral carotid or occipital artery (if the latter vessel is a known feeder to the fistula) is performed for 30 minutes at a time, three times a day. If compression of the carotid artery is chosen, patients are instructed to use the contralateral arm.
- In 25 % of simple DAVFs of the transverse/sigmoid sinuses supplied by the occipital artery, compression of the occipital artery results in complete thrombosis of the DAVF within several weeks.
- The Borden classification system stratifies lesions on the basis of the site of venous drainage and the presence or absence of cortical venous drainage.

✅ **Borden classification**
- **Type I:**
  - Drainage into a meningeal vein, spinal epidural veins, or into a dural venous sinus
  - Normal anterograde flow in both the draining veins and other veins draining into the system

- Usually have benign clinical behavior with a favorable natural history
- Equivalent to Cognard type I and IIa
- **Type II:**
  - Drainage into meningeal veins, spinal epidural veins, or into a dural venous sinus
  - Retrograde flow into the normal subarachnoid veins
  - It may present with hemorrhage due to venous hypertension
  - Equivalent to Cognard types IIb and IIa+b
- **Type III:**
  - Direct drainage into subarachnoid veins or into an isolated segment of the venous sinus
  - Retrograde flow into the normal cortical veins
  - Results from a thrombosis on either side of the dural sinus segment and will cause venous hypertension with a risk of hemorrhage
  - Equivalent to Cognard types III, IV, and V

✅ According to this classification, these lesions are further subclassified into **type a** (single hole) or **type b** (multiple hole) fistulas.

❓ 11. **DAVFs**
Borden classification, the FALSE answer is:
   A. Type III fistulas have both anterograde venous sinus drainage and retrograde drainage into subarachnoid veins.
   B. In type III fistulas, the venous sinus is always closed.
   C. In type III fistulas, high-flow venopathy causes reversal of flow into the arterialized leptomeningeal veins.
   D. Type III fistulas have exclusive retrograde drainage into arterialized subarachnoid veins at/or on the wall of dural venous sinuses.
   E. In type III fistulas, when the sinus is patent, the point of the fistula can be located between the meningeal artery and leptomeningeal vein.

✅ The answer is **B.**
- In type III fistulas, the venous sinus may be patent but largely defunctionalized because of high-flow venopathy causing reversal of flow into arterialized leptomeningeal veins.
- In type III fistulas, when the sinus is patent, the point of the fistula is located either between the meningeal artery and leptomeningeal vein or between the meningeal artery and a segment of arterialized dural venous sinus that is thrombosed at either end or somehow isolated from the rest of the sinus, thereby causing reversal of drainage into leptomeningeal veins.

? 12. DAVFs

Cognard classification, the FALSE answer is:

A. Type I fistulas, located in the main sinus, with antegrade flow
B. Type II fistulas, in the main sinus, with reflux into the sinus, cortical veins, or both
C. Type III fistulas with direct cortical venous drainage with venous ectasia
D. Type IV fistulas with direct cortical venous drainage with venous ectasia
E. Type V fistulas with spinal venous drainage

✓ The answer is **C**.

- Type III with direct cortical venous drainage without venous ectasia
- Type II fistulas, in the main sinus, with reflux into the sinus (IIa), cortical veins (IIb), or both (IIa+b)
- The Cognard classification is based on angiographic patterns and is generally more applicable to DAVFs involving the transverse sinus.
- **The Cognard classification** divides dural arteriovenous fistulas into 5 types according to the following features:
  - Location of fistula
  - Presence of cortical venous drainage
  - Direction of flow
  - Presence of venous ectasia
- **Cognard classification system:**
  - **Type I:**
    - Confined to sinus
    - Antegrade flow
    - No cortical venous drainage/reflux
  - **Type II:**
    - IIa:
      - Confined to sinus
      - Retrograde flow (reflux) into sinus
      - No cortical venous drainage/reflux
    - IIb:
      - Drains into sinus with reflux into cortical veins
      - Antegrade flow
    - IIa+b:
      - Drains into sinus with reflux into cortical veins
      - Retrograde flow
  - **Type III:**
    - Drains directly into cortical veins (not into sinus) drainage (40 % hemorrhage)

- **Type IV:**
  - Drains directly into cortical veins (not into sinus) drainage with venous ectasia (65 % hemorrhage)
- **Type V:**
  - Spinal perimedullary venous drainage associated with progressive myelopathy

13. DAVFs
Treatment, the FALSE answer is:
A. Indications for intervention include neurologic dysfunction, hemorrhage, and refractory symptoms.
B. For the treatment to be complete, external carotid injections must demonstrate no abnormal AV shunting.
C. Most DAVFs are better treated endovascularly.
D. Placement copious dural tack-up sutures should be avoided as it predisposes to subdural hematoma.
E. The use of the craniotome is discouraged, as a sinus or venous laceration could produce a fatal hemorrhage.

The answer is **D.**
- Extra care is taken to place copious dural tack-up sutures to obliterate the epidural space which is abnormally vascular.
- Most DAVFs are better treated endovascularly; however, ethmoidal DAVFs are probably best treated microsurgically.

14. DAVFs
Treatment, the FALSE answer is:
A. Treatment modalities for DAVFs include resection, embolization, and radiosurgery.
B. Radiosurgery should be reserved for benign DAVFs that have failed other treatments.
C. Radiosurgery is expected to cause obliteration of DAVFs 1–3 years after the procedure
D. Typically, radiosurgery is performed after embolization.
E. Radiosurgery must ensure that the entire fistula is included in the irradiated volume.

The answer is **D.**
- Typically, radiosurgery is performed before any embolization to ensure that the entire fistula is included in the irradiated volume.

? 15. **DAVFs**

Treatment, the FALSE answer is:

A. Currently, initial treatment of most DAVFs involves endovascular techniques.

B. DAVFs of the tentorium are traditionally difficult to obliterate endovascularly.

C. DAVFs of the tentorium have multiple small feeding arteries, which are hard to visualize and often originate off the ICAs.

D. Trans-arterial embolization reduces flow through the fistula and can produce complete thrombosis of the DAVF 60 % of the time.

E. Transvenous treatment is appropriate for a Cognard type III fistula, in which there is drainage into the sinus and then reflux into a cortical vein.

✓ The answer is **E.**

- Transvenous treatment is appropriate for a Cognard type IIb fistula, in which there is drainage into the sinus and then reflux into a cortical vein. But it is not appropriate for a Cognard type III fistula, in which there is drainage into a cortical vein and then the sinus.

- Transvenous embolization has been advocated as the preferred endovascular treatment route because of higher occlusion rates, fewer complications, and a lower rate of recanalization than with trans-arterial embolization.

- In the latter case, transvenous occlusion of the sinus blocks eventual venous egress, thus further elevating pressure in the arterialized subarachnoid vein.

- Although generally viewed as incomplete treatment, trans-arterial embolization to reduce flow through the fistula has been reported to produce complete thrombosis of the DAVF 60 % of the time.

? 16. **DAVFs**

Treatment, the FALSE answer is:

A. Microsurgery is the primary modality of treatment for persistent cortical venous drainage following maximal endovascular therapy.

B. Arterial feeders are coagulated and the leptomeningeal arterialized veins are then occluded and divided as close to their dural origin as possible.

C. DAVFs occur more common in children, and when they do they tend to be simple.

D. May be associated with neurofibromatosis type 1.

E. Cerebral aneurysms can be associated with DAVFs, especially those located in the anterior cranial fossa and the convexities.

✓ The answer is **C**.

- While congenital DAVFs may rarely occur in children and are typically more complex than adult DAVFs, the majority of adult DAVFs are considered to be acquired idiopathic lesions.
- The approach to pediatric patients with congenital DAVFs and congestive heart failure involves diminution of flow to permit survival and growth, usually by trans-arterial or mixed trans-arterial/transvenous techniques.
- If residual DAVF is present, cure is attempted at a later date (3 to 6 months of age). DAVFs occur rarely in children, and when they do they tend to be complex and bilateral.
- DAVFs may be associated with Ehlers-Danlos syndrome, fibromuscular dysplasia, or neurofibromatosis type 1.

? 17. **DAVFs**

Transverse-sigmoid sinus DAVFs, the FALSE answer is:
A. Account for 62 % of the DAVFs.
B. Nearly half of these patients had a cranial bruit.
C. Never caused by sigmoid sinus occlusion.
D. The occipital artery is the dominant feeder in most cases.
E. Treatment is recommended for all symptomatic transverse-sigmoid sinuses.

✓ The answer is **C**.

- May be caused by sigmoid sinus occlusion, possibly from chronic infection or trauma.
- Nearly half of these patients had a cranial bruit because of proximity of the draining sinus to the middle ear.
- Treatment is recommended for all symptomatic transverse-sigmoid sinuses; transvenous embolization is the favored approach, if technically feasible.

? 18. **DAVFs***

Tentorial DAVFs, the FALSE answer is:
A. Account for 12 % of DAVFs.
B. The initial symptoms are tinnitus in 70 % to 88 %.
C. Rarely shows aggressive clinical symptoms.
D. Usually drains to junction of transverse and sigmoid sinuses but almost not more than 1 cm from the junction.
E. The treatment in general is similar to other locations.

✅ The answer is **C.**
- Show aggressive symptoms in 92 % of cases.
- Arterial feeders are derived from the meningo-hypophyseal trunk, occipital artery, ascending pharyngeal artery, and vertebral artery.

❓ 19. DAVFs*

Superior sagittal sinus DAVFs, the FALSE answer is:
- A. Account for 8 % of the DAVFs.
- B. Has female predominance.
- C. Feeders are most commonly from the ICA.
- D. Usually retrograde drainage into the parasagittal cortical veins.
- E. Trans-arterial embolization and surgical coagulation of the draining vein are the preferred treatment options.

✅ The answer is **C.**
- Treatment is often challenging because of multiple and bilateral arterial feeders, most commonly the middle meningeal arteries.
- 50 % of patients have headache.

❓ 20. DAVFs*

Anterior fossa DAVFs, the FALSE answer is:
- A. Anterior fossa DAVFs located at the cribriform plate at the level of the foramen cecum.
- B. Anterior fossa DAVFs are more common in males unlike other locations.
- C. The usual presentation is stroke.
- D. Supplied by ethmoidal branches of the ophthalmic arteries.
- E. Surgery is an excellent option.

✅ The answer is **C.**
- Anterior fossa DAVFs are nearly always symptomatic with the usual presentation is SAH.

❓ 21. DAVFs*

The FALSE answer is:
- A. Foramen magnum DAVFs are usually presented with progressive myelopathy.
- B. Foramen magnum DAVFs usually cause venous hypertension of the spinal cord.
- C. Foramen magnum DAVFs arterial feeders are from the occipital arteries, ICA, and vertebral arteries.

D. Torcular Herophili DAVFs very rarely have aggressive neurological symptoms.
E. Cavernous sinus DAVFs account for 10–15 % of DAVFs, with treatment is necessary.

✓ The answer is **D**.
- Torcular Herophili DAVFs always have aggressive neurological symptoms.
- Foramen magnum DAVFs are usually presented with progressive myelopathy in 50 % of patients.

3.2   Carotid-Cavernous Fistula

❓ 22. Carotid-cavernous fistula (CCF)
Definition, the FALSE answer is:
A. An abnormal communication between the ICA or one of its branches or the ECA and the cavernous sinus (CS).
B. The most common cause for the development of CCFs is trauma.
C. The most common complications associated with CCFs involve the ocular findings.
D. Usually CCF occurs in infancy.
E. The two main trunks of the cavernous ICA are commonly implicated in CCFs.

✓ The answer is **D**.
- Usually CCF occurs in the middle aged, but can occur in childhood or infancy.
- The two main trunks of the cavernous ICA, both commonly implicated in dural CCFs, are the meningo-hypophyseal trunk (most constant) and the inferolateral trunk.

❓ 23. CCF
Cavernous sinus (CS) surgical anatomy, the FALSE answer is:
A. CS is an extradurally located sinus.
B. The most constant branch of cavernous ICA is the meningo-hypophyseal trunk.
C. The CS in direct continuity through the clivus with the epidural space surrounding the spine.
D. The inferior hypophyseal artery arises directly from cavernous ICA.
E. There are constant anastomoses between branches of the ICA and the ECA. Although not always angiographically visible.

✅ The answer is **D**.
- The inferior hypophyseal artery arises from the meningo-hypophyseal trunk of the cavernous ICA.
- Anatomically, cavernous sinus is an extradurally located sinus, whereas other dural sinuses are located between two dural walls in the cranial cavity.
- CS is an extradural space between the two layers of dura laterally and superiorly and the periosteum of lateral portion of the sphenoid bone inferiorly and medially.
- The ICA with its dural branches traverses the cavernous sinus along with cranial nerves III, IV, V, and VI.
- The two main trunks of the cavernous ICA, both commonly implicated in dural CCFs, are the meningo-hypophyseal trunk (most constant) and the inferolateral trunk.
- The meningo-hypophyseal trunk originates near the posterior genu and gives three branches: (i) the tentorial artery, (ii) the dorsal meningeal (clival) artery, and (iii) the inferior hypophyseal artery.
- The inferolateral trunk originates laterally near the middle of the horizontal segment, courses over the abducent nerve, supplies the adjacent cavernous sinus dura and cranial nerves, and commonly anastomoses with the maxillary and/or middle meningeal arteries through the artery of the foramen rotundum, the artery of the foramen ovale, and/or the foramen spinosum.
- McConnell's capsular arteries are inconstant medial branches to the pituitary originating more anteriorly from the horizontal segment of the cavernous ICA.

❓ **24. CCF**
Cavernous sinus surgical anatomy, the FALSE answer is:
A. Cavernous sinus is a single venous cavity.
B. The anterior portion receives ophthalmic veins and the sphenoparietal sinus.
C. Posterior drainage is through the basilar plexus and the petrosal sinuses.
D. Inferolaterally, connections exist through dural veins draining into the pterygoid plexus.
E. The two cavernous sinuses communicate through the anterior and posterior intercavernous sinus forming a circular sinus.

✅ The answer is **A**.
- Cavernous sinus is not a single venous space, but exhibits compartmentalization that contains a plexiform arrangement of the veins.
- The oculomotor nerve is located within the superior lateral cavernous sinus wall and courses anteriorly just beneath the ACP to enter the orbit through the SOF.
- The trochlear nerve is also located within the lateral cavernous sinus wall, traveling just beneath and parallel to the oculomotor nerve.
- The first division of the trigeminal nerve (V1) courses several millimeters below the oculomotor and trochlear nerves within the lateral sinus wall, whereas the abducent nerve courses within the cavernous venous compartment between the cavernous segment and V1.
- Finally, sympathetic fiber bundles course as a plexus along the cavernous and clinoidal ICA, eventually departing the ICA proximal to the dural ring to project into the orbit.
- Disruption of these fibers can occur from operative manipulation of the clinoidal segment, causing mild postoperative ptosis or miosis without facial anhidrosis.

❓ 25. **CCF**
   Types, the FALSE answer is:
   A. Type A is direct high-flow shunt between ICA and cavernous sinus.
   B. Type B is indirect low-flow shunt from meningeal branches of ICA.
   C. Type C is indirect low-flow shunt from meningeal branches of ECA.
   D. Type D is indirect low-flow shunt from meningeal branches of both ICA and ECA.
   E. Type D is the most common type.

✅ The answer is **E**.
- Type A is the most common type.
- Type D is the most common low flow.
- They are based on angiographic features (high-flow and low-flow fistulas), mechanism of onset (spontaneous and traumatic), morphology, and angioarchitecture (direct and indirect fistulas).
- CCF are divided by Barrow classification into direct (type A) and indirect (types B–D) based on arterial supply.
- Direct (type A) CCF can be subdivided into: A1, direct CCF only or A2, direct CCF with an aneurysm.
- Type B is extremely rare.

Barrow classification of CCFs		
Type	Fistulous vessel	Comments
A	From ICA to CS	Direct, high flow, the most common
B	Dural ICA branches to CS: Meningo-hypophyseal trunk (66 %) Inferolateral trunk (30 %)	Indirect, low flow
C	ECA branches to CS: Internal maxillary (67 %) Middle meningeal (59 %) Accessory meningeal (31 %) Ascending pharyngeal (24 %)	Indirect, low flow
D	Both ICA and ECA branches	Indirect, low flow, the most common low flow

	Direct CCF	Indirect CCF
Arterial source	Tear in the cavernous ICA	ICA/ECA meningeal branches
Etiology	Often traumatic	Spontaneous
Population	Young male	Elderly female
Hemodynamic behavior	High flow	Low flow
Clinical presentation	Dramatic and rapid	Subtle and slowly progressive
Spontaneous resolution	Uncommon	Common

26. CCF

Types, the FALSE answer is:

A. All types are supplied by the ECA except type A and B.

B. All types are supplied by the ICA except type C.

C. Indirect (dural) are low-flow shunts from dural branches of ECA (not from ICA) except type B.

D. Patients with indirect CCFs never have bilateral involvement.

E. Indirect CCFs are much more frequent in females.

✅ The answer is **D**.
- Up to 19 % of patients with indirect CCFs have bilateral involvement.

❓ **27. CCF**
   Traumatic CCFs, the FALSE answer is:
   A. Traumatic CCFs are the most common type.
   B. Traumatic CCFs are usually of high flow.
   C. Traumatic CCFs occur in 0.2 % of head injury.
   D. Traumatic CCFs occur in 4 % of basilar skull fractures.
   E. Traumatic CCFs are more common after penetrating head injury.

✅ The answer is **E**.
- Traumatic CCFs are more common after closed head injury, but can result from penetrating trauma to the head that result in injury to the cavernous ICA.
- Direct CCFs can be divided into traumatic (70 % to 90 %) and spontaneous.

❓ **28. CCF**
   Causes of iatrogenic CCFs, the FALSE answer is:
   A. Craniotomy
   B. Carotid endarterectomy
   C. Transsphenoidal/sinus surgery
   D. Microvascular decompression of trigeminal nerve
   E. Endovascular procedures

✅ The answer is **D**.
- Iatrogenic may be due to craniotomy, carotid endarterectomy, transsphenoidal/sinus surgery, endovascular procedures, or **percutaneous trigeminal rhizotomy**.

❓ **29. CCF**
   Spontaneous CCFs, the FALSE answer is:
   A. Spontaneous CCFs account for 30 % of CCF.
   B. Spontaneous fistulas are mostly high flow.
   C. The most common cause of spontaneous CCF is rupture of cavernous ICA aneurysm.
   D. Spontaneous CCFs may occur in Ehlers-Danlos syndrome or fibromuscular dysplasia.
   E. Spontaneous CCFs may develop following pregnancy, sinusitis, or resolution of cavernous sinus thrombosis.

✅ The answer is **B**.
- Spontaneous fistulas are mostly low flow and account for 20–30 % of CCF.
- Spontaneous CCFs occur in up to 24 % of individuals with cavernous ICA aneurysm.

❓ **30. CCF**
Clinical features, the FALSE answer is:
A. The classic triad is chemosis, pulsatile proptosis, and ocular bruit.
B. Classic triad is more common with indirect CCF.
C. The most common initial presentation of direct CCFs is orbital bruit.
D. Proptosis is common in initial presentation of direct CCFs up to 72 % of patients.
E. Indirect CCFs generally have a more gradual onset and milder presentation than direct.

✅ The answer is **B**.
- Classic triad is more common with direct CCF.
- The most common initial presentation of direct CCFs is orbital bruit (80 %) and proptosis (72 %).

❓ **31. CCF**
Clinical features, the FALSE answer is:
A. Traumatic CCFs occur mostly in older age group.
B. Spontaneous CCFs occur in the older age group.
C. Indirect CCFs are common in older age group.
D. Spontaneous CCFs have a female predominance.
E. Spontaneous CCFs may have a male predominance.

✅ The answer is **A**.
- Traumatic CCF occurs mostly in young age with a suggested male predominance.
- Indirect CCFs are commonly encountered in the sixth and seventh decades of life (mean age, 66.8 years).
- Spontaneous fistulas occur in the older age group with a female preponderance (7:1 female-to-male ratio).

❓ **32. CCF**
Clinical features, the FALSE answer is:
A. Ocular and/or cranial bruit.
B. If the intraocular pressure is very high, the bruit may not be heard.

C. Diplopia is most commonly due to oculomotor nerve palsy.
D. Ophthalmoplegia is usually unilateral.
E. Secondary open-angle glaucoma.

✓ The answer is **C**.
  − Diplopia is most commonly due to abducent nerve palsy.
  − Deterioration of visual acuity may be due to hypoxic retinopathy as a result of reduced arterial pressure and increased venous pressure and increased intraocular pressure.
  − Neovascularization of the iris or retina can also occur.
  − Ophthalmoplegia (usually unilateral, but may present initially as bilateral or may progress to bilateral).
  − CCF also may show central retinal vein occlusion → secondary open-angle glaucoma.
  − The bruit disappears on compression of the carotid in the neck.

❓ 33. **CCF**
   Clinical features, the FALSE answer is:
   A. Posteriorly placed fistulas mostly have a significant exophthalmic component.
   B. Life-threatening epistaxis is not uncommon with a traumatic direct CCF.
   C. ICH can occur with both direct and indirect fistulas associated with retrograde cortical venous drainage.
   D. ICH in the setting of a direct CCF frequently portends a poor prognosis.
   E. CCFs rarely cause SAH.

✓ The answer is **A**.
  − Anteriorly placed fistulas mostly have a significant exophthalmic component.
  − Posterior placed fistulas often have contralateral involvement.
  − Epistaxis, even life-threatening epistaxis, is not uncommon with a traumatic direct CCF and can occur weeks after the trauma.
  − The CCFs that drain posteriorly into the superior and inferior petrosal sinuses are usually asymptomatic.
  − Those which drain into supratentorial cortical or posterior fossa veins often present as intracerebral hemorrhage due to rupture of arterialized veins.
  − Those which drain into pterygoid plexus of veins may be asymptomatic or cause pain in the maxillary or mandibular area.
  − ICH in the setting of a direct CCF frequently portends a poor prognosis with a high risk for short-term rehemorrhage.

? **34. CCF**
Radiology, the FALSE answer is:
A. The serpiginous and engorged superior ophthalmic vein is common sign in CT and MRI.
B. T2WI coronal helps to differentiate superior ophthalmic vein from rectus muscles.
C. The engorged superior ophthalmic vein sign is not present in cavernous meningioma.
D. CT and MRI may also help to study the extent of skull fracture in traumatic CCFs.
E. CT and MRI may show an enlarged cavernous sinus with a convex shape to the lateral wall.

✓ The answer is **C.**
- Serpiginous and engorged intraocular vessels especially the superior ophthalmic vein (best seen on T2WI coronal, helps to differentiate from rectus muscles). However, this sign may also be present in orbital pseudotumor, cavernous meningioma and Grave's ophthalmopathy.
- CT and MRI show enlarged superior ophthalmic vein (usually > 4 mm), enlarged muscles, and enlarged cavernous sinus with a convex shape to the lateral wall may suggest a CCF.
- In MRI the CCF may appear as Caput medusa (engorged, serpiginous intraocular vessels) on T2.

? **35. CCF**
Radiology, the FALSE answer is:
A. The definitive study to diagnose a CCF is digital subtraction angiography.
B. Huber maneuver of angiography helps to identify lower extent of fistula.
C. Mehringer-Hieshima maneuver of angiography includes injecting the affected ICA while gently compressing the CCA of the neck.
D. Selective injection of the external carotid system is important to define the supply and angioarchitecture of indirect CCFs.
E. Low-flow indirect CCFs may not be visualized on CCA injections only.

✓ The answer is **B.**
- Huber maneuver of angiography: lateral view, inject vertebral artery and manually compress affected carotid. Helps identify upper extent of fistula, multiple fistulous openings, and complete transection of ICA.

- The definitive study and gold standard to diagnose a CCF is digital subtraction angiography.
- Definitive diagnosis is based on catheter angiography, which must include selective injections of both ICAs and ECAs and at least one vertebral artery. Low-flow indirect CCFs may not be visualized on CCA injections only.

❓ 36. CCF
   Treatment (noninvasive), the FALSE answer is:
   A. Medical management is reserved for treatment of low-risk indirect CCFs with ocular findings.
   B. An old-aged patient with Barrow type C fistula would most likely be a candidate for an initial trial of nonoperative treatment.
   C. Carotid self-compression therapy can be attempted as a noninvasive treatment in low-risk cases.
   D. Manual compression therapy can occlude indirect CCFs in about 75 % of cases.
   E. The contralateral hand is used to compress the carotid artery in the neck for brief periods of time several times per day.

✅ The answer is D.
- Manual compression therapy can occlude indirect CCFs in about 30 % of cases (20–50 % or 10 to 60 % in some texts), therefore one may observe these as long as visual acuity is stable and intraocular pressure is < 25.
- Carotid self-compression (manual) therapy to assist with spontaneous thrombosis of the CCFs can be attempted as a noninvasive treatment in low-risk cases.
- Carotid self-compression is done for 20–30 seconds 4 times per hour for 4 to 6 weeks. Patient is instructed to compress carotid artery on the side of the lesion using contralateral hand (should patient develop cerebral ischemia during compression, contralateral hand likely will be affected, releasing compression).
- Prism glasses or patching for diplopia, topical medications for increased intraocular pressures, and lubrication to minimize risk of proptosis-related keratopathy.

❓ 37. CCF
   Treatment (indications for early treatment), the FALSE answer is:
   A. Spontaneous closure from thrombosis of cavernous sinus is unlikely.
   B. Bruit.

C. Disfiguring progressive proptosis causing exposure keratopathy.
D. Progressive visual failure.
E. Early filling of cortical veins on angiography.

✓ The answer is **B**.
- Intolerable bruit.
- Other indications for early treatment of CCFs are glaucoma, intolerable headache, diplopia, SAH, ICH, or extension into air sinus.
- Symptomatic high-flow CCFs rarely resolve spontaneously, and urgent treatment is usually indicated.
- Spontaneous closure from thrombosis of cavernous sinus is unlikely (as in trauma, high flow).
- Treatment is usually in the form of endovascular embolization or trapping between surgically placed clips.

❓ 38. CCF
Treatment, the FALSE answer is:
A. The long-term occlusion rate for endovascular treatment of CCFs is 76–100 %.
B. A direct CCF should be considered for endovascular treatment via trans-arterial and/or transvenous approach.
C. Indirect CCFs that fail conservative treatment should be considered for endovascular treatment.
D. Endovascular treatment is necessary if the parent artery is damaged.
E. Surgery may involve ligation of the common or internal carotid artery if embolization fails.

✓ The answer is **D**.
- Surgical treatment can be necessary if the parent artery is particularly damaged and concern exists regarding catheterization of a disrupted vessel, in which case trapping of the damaged segment and the fistula is a valid option.

❓ 39. CCF
Endovascular treatment, the FALSE answer is:
A. Onyx has become the mainstay of treatment of direct CCFs.
B. Routes include transvenous via superior ophthalmic vein or through petrosal sinus to cavernous sinus.
C. Routes include trans-arterial through ICA or ECA.

D. Trans-arterial embolization is reserved for ruptured cavernous ICA aneurysms in direct CCFs.

E. Trans-arterial embolization is reserved for ruptured meningeal feeders of the ECA in indirect CCFs.

✅ The answer is **A**.
- Detachable coils have become the mainstay of treatment of direct CCFs.
- Unlike coils, which may further compartmentalize the CS, onyx tends to more fully obliterate the fistulous connection.
- The main advantage of detachable coils is their ability to be retrieved in the event of inadequate placement.
- A trans-arterial approach to indirect CCFs can be used when adequate supply from the external carotid branches exists.
- Routes available include trans-arterial through ICA or ECA (useful only for dural fistulas).
- If trans-arterial embolization fails (e.g., wide aneurysm neck), the carotid artery may be occluded on either side of fistula to trap it (sacrifices carotid artery, therefore test occlusion must be done first to determine if patient can tolerate this). The distal occlusion needs to be proximal to the ophthalmic artery.

❓ **40. CCF***
Transvenous endovascular treatment, the FALSE answer is:
A. TVE has higher success rate than trans-arterial route.
B. TVE should not be used for treatment of Barrow type B CCFs.
C. TVE may be used to treat traumatic direct CCFs or type C or D CCFs as well.
D. TVE can be done via traversing the heart to enter the jugular vein and then pass through the petrosal sinus to cavernous sinus.
E. TVE can be done via supraorbital vein while enters orbit to become superior ophthalmic vein.

✅ The answer is **A**.
- TVE has lower success rate (20 %) than trans-arterial route.
- Transvenous embolization is the primary treatment of Barrow type B CCFs because of the risk of reflux of embolizate into the ICA.
- Transvenous via superior ophthalmic vein: must avoid lacerating the vein inside the orbit and avoid distal ligation of the vein without proximal occlusion (shunts even more blood into the eye).

- In TVE via superior ophthalmic vein, it is best to wait for the vein to become arterialized by the high-flow pressure.
- The surgeon should strike a balance between packing the sinus enough to occlude the fistula and over packing, which can cause cranial nerve palsies.

(?) 41. CCF*

Radiosurgery treatment, the FALSE answer is:
- A. An effective treatment of direct CCFs.
- B. The drawback is latency time during which there is potential risk for ICH.
- C. The rationale for performing embolization after radiosurgery is to allow adequate coverage of the fistulous nidus without having it obscured by the embolization.
- D. Trans-arterial particle embolization can decrease the flow to lesion while radiosurgery takes effect.
- E. With combined radiosurgery and embolization, chemosis and proptosis improved in 94 %.

(✓) The answer is A.
- Radiosurgery is an effective treatment of low-flow indirect CCFs.
- The drawback of radiosurgery is the latency time during which patients continue to be exposed to the symptoms and the potential for intracranial hemorrhage.
- With combined radiosurgery and embolization strategy, chemosis and proptosis were improved in 94 % and 88 % experienced resolution of their visual symptoms.

(?) 42. CCF*

Morbidity and mortality, the FALSE answer is:
- A. Mortality associated with CCFs is due to retrograde cortical drainage resulting in venous congestion and hemorrhages.
- B. Complication rate is up to 10 % with multimodality endovascular treatment.
- C. Complication rate is generally higher for indirect CCFs.
- D. Paradoxical aggravation of the ocular symptoms is uncommon.
- E. Recurrence rate of CCF in general is 1–4 %.

✓ The answer is **C**.
- Complication rates are generally higher for direct CCFs.
- Following treatment, complication rates are up to 10 % with multimodality endovascular treatment.
- Paradoxical aggravation of the ocular symptoms is uncommon (3 %) and probably related to the effects of CS thrombosis or mass effect from the embolizing material.
- Up to a third of patients show worsening of preexisting or new extraocular motility deficits after detachable balloon treatment. Often due to the compression of the sixth cranial nerve running in the CS, usually transient.

Cavernoma and Other Malformations

This book contains some difficult questions marked with " * " sign.

© Springer International Publishing AG 2017
S.S. Hoz, *Vascular Neurosurgery*, DOI 10.1007/978-3-319-49187-5_4

? 1. Cavernoma (cavernous malformation, cavernous hemangioma, or cavernous angioma)
The FALSE answer is:
A. A low-flow well-circumscribed, benign vascular hamartoma.
B. Cavernomas consist of irregular thick- and thin-walled sinusoidal vascular channels located within the brain but no arteries.
C. Cavernomas comprise 9 % of CNS vascular malformations.
D. Cavernomas are mainly supratentorial.
E. Cavernomas are the only vascular malformation with intervening neural parenchyma.

✓ The answer is **E**.
  — The only vascular malformation **without** intervening neural parenchyma.
  — A low-flow well-circumscribed, benign vascular hamartoma consisting of irregular thick- and thinwalled sinusoidal channels located within the brain but no arteries.

? 2. Cavernomas
Location, the FALSE answer is:
A. Two-thirds are supratentorial.
B. Common in the frontal or temporal lobes.
C. 4–35 % of cavernomas in the brainstem.
D. 5–10 % of cavernomas in the basal ganglia.
E. Associated with developmental venous anomaly (DVA) that should be resected also.

✓ The answer is **E**.
  — Associated with DVA (represents venous outflow and should be preserved).
  — 4–35 % of cavernomas in the brainstem (commonly in the pons).

? 3. Cavernoma
Pathology, the FALSE answer is:
A. Caverns are filled with blood in various stages of thrombus formation, organization, and dissolution and may calcify.
B. Cavernoma's gross appearance resembles a mulberry.
C. Cavernoma is sometimes called "the hemorrhoid of the brain."
D. Cavernoma has abnormally hypertrophied smooth muscle layer.
E. Two types: sporadic and hereditary (autosomal dominant).

✅ The answer is **D**.
 ⁼ Smooth muscle layer is absent or minimum.
 ⁼ Light microscopy: stains for von Willebrand's factor.
 ⁼ EM: shows abnormal gapping of the tight junctions between endothelial cells (may permit leakage of blood).

❓ 4. **Cavernoma***
   Pathology, the FALSE answer is:
   A. Cystic variant of cavernoma occurs more commonly in the posterior fossa.
   B. Dural-based variant of cavernoma occurs more commonly in the parasellar area.
   C. Hemangioma calcificans variant of cavernoma occurs more in the temporal lobe.
   D. Cavernomas are very rarely multiple.
   E. Previous radiotherapy appears to be a risk factor.

✅ The answer is **D**.
 ⁼ Cavernomas are multiple in less than 50 %.
 ⁼ Previous radiotherapy appears to be a risk factor especially for spinal cavernomas.

❓ 5. **Cavernoma**
   Presentation, the FALSE answer is:
   A. The most common presentation is seizures and progressive neurologic deficit.
   B. 20 % of cavernomas presented with hemorrhage.
   C. Hemorrhage appears to be higher in females.
   D. Hemorrhage is always fatal.
   E. Cavernoma may rarely present with hydrocephalus or as in incidental finding.

✅ The answer is **D**.
 ⁼ Hemorrhage risk is difficult to predict, but rarely fatal.
 ⁼ The common presentations are seizures (60 %), progressive neurologic deficit (50 %), hemorrhage (20 %) (usually intraparenchymal), hydrocephalus, or as in incidental finding.

? **6. Cavernoma**
Risk factors for hemorrhage, the FALSE answer is:
A. The size of the cavernoma (>1 cm)
B. Female gender and pregnancy
C. Prior symptomatic bleed
D. Age more than 35 years
E. Deep location of the lesion

✓ The answer is **D**.
— Age less than 35 years is also a risk factor for hemorrhage.

? **7. Cavernoma**
Radiology, the FALSE answer is:
A. CT scan is sensitive but not specific.
B. Gradient-echo T2WI MRI is the most sensitive test.
C. In MRI, the mixed signal core with low-signal rim described as "popcorn" pattern is pathognomonic.
D. Angiography is highly sensitive for cavernomas.
E. The diagnosis is strongly suggested by finding multiple lesions with a positive family history.

✓ The answer is **D**.
— Angiography for cavernomas is usually negative (usually angiographically occult).
— CT scan is sensitive but not specific. May overlap with low-grade tumors, hemorrhages, and granulomas.
— Diffusion tensor imaging/white matter tractography and preop 3D-constructive interference in steady-state (CISS) MRI may improve localization, approach, and post-op outcomes.

? **8. Cavernoma***
Radiology, Zabramski classification, the FALSE answer is:
A. Type I: subacute hemorrhage
B. Type II: classic "popcorn ball" lesion
C. Type III: chronic hemorrhage
D. Type IV: multiple punctate micro-hemorrhages
E. Type I is the most common type

✅ The answer is **E**.
- Type **II** is the most common type.
- The **Zabramski classification** is a radiological **classification of cerebral cavernomas** malformations.
  Zabramski classification of cavernomas:
  - **Type I**: subacute hemorrhage
    - T1: hyperintense
    - T2: hypo- or hyperintense
  - **Type II**: most common type—classic "popcorn" lesion
    - T1: mixed signal intensity centrally
    - T2: mixed signal intensity centrally
    - Low-signal rim with blooming on T2 sequences
  - **Type III**: chronic hemorrhage
    - T1: hypointense to isointense centrally
    - T2: hypointense centrally
    - Low-signal rim with blooming on T2 sequences
  - **Type IV**: multiple punctate micro-hemorrhages
    - T1: difficult to identify
    - T2: difficult to identify
    - T2 gradient echo: "black dots" with blooming
    - Difficult to distinguish from small capillary telangiectasias

❓ 9. **Cavernoma**
   Indications of surgery, the FALSE answer is:
   A. Accessible lesions with focal deficit
   B. Less accessible lesions that repeatedly bleed with progressive neurologic deterioration may be considered for excision
   C. Brainstem cavernomas that have not bled
   D. Symptomatic hemorrhage
   E. New onset seizures or difficult to manage seizures

✅ The answer is **C**.
- Surgery is almost never indicated for brainstem cavernomas that have not bled.

❓ 10. **Cavernoma**
   Management, the FALSE answer is:
   A. Asymptomatic, incidentally discovered cavernomas should be managed expectantly.
   B. Expectant management is usually with serial imaging studies for about 2–3 years.

    C. Never remove the hemosiderin-stained brain immediately surrounding the cavernoma.
    D. Goal of surgery is complete removal of the malformation.
    E. Piecemeal excision is an option, especially in brainstem cavernomas.

✅ The answer is **C**.
- For supratentorial cavernomas presenting with seizures, it is desirable to also remove the hemosiderin-stained brain immediately surrounding the cavernoma.
- Expectant management is usually with serial imaging studies for about 2–3 years (to rule out frequent subclinical bleeds).

❓ 11. **Cavernoma**
    Management, the FALSE answer is:
    A. If an associated venous angioma is found, it should not be removed.
    B. Biopsy to verify the diagnosis is usually indicated.
    C. Stereotactic radiosurgery is not an alternative to surgery.
    D. Outcome is worse with surgery through the floor of the fourth ventricle than with a lateral approach.
    E. Worsening of neurologic outcome is more in deep cavernoma resections than in superficial.

✅ The answer is **B**.
- Since the radiographic appearance is almost pathognomonic, biopsy to verify the diagnosis is rarely appropriate.
- If an associated venous angioma is found, it should not be removed as they represent the venous drainage of the area.
- Worsening of neurologic outcome was 9 % vs. 29 % in superficial vs. deep brainstem cavernoma resections, respectively.

4.1   Developmental Venous Anomaly

❓ 12. **DVA, developmental venous anomaly or venous malformation or venous angioma**
    General, the FALSE answer is:
    A. DVA is not a pathologic lesion, but a normal variant.
    B. DVA has several prominent deep parenchymal veins that drain a normal part of the brain and then drain into an unusually large draining vein.

C. Pathologic characteristics consist of anomalous veins separated by normal brain tissue.
D. DVAs are high-flow, high-pressure lesions.
E. There is an equal prevalence in men and women.

✅ The answer is **D**.
- DVAs are low-flow, low-pressure lesions.

❓ 13. **DVA**
Presentation, the FALSE answer is:
A. DVAs are the most common intracranial vascular malformation in autopsy.
B. DVAs are the least common form encountered in surgical series.
C. Most are clinically silent.
D. DVAs are most commonly seen in the occipital lobe.
E. Most common in regions supplied by the MCA.

✅ The answer is **D**.
- DVAs are commonly seen in the frontal lobe or in the cerebellum.
- The diagnosis is typically made in the third decade.
- Rarely cause seizures and even less frequently hemorrhage may occur.
- Most common in regions supplied by the MCA or in the region of vein of Galen.

❓ 14. **DVA**
Radiology, the FALSE answer is:
A. The angiographic and MRI appearance is pathognomonic resembling the "head of Medusa."
B. The "head of Medusa" sign has other names like a hydra or a spider.
C. In angiography, the DVA appears as a long draining vein (longer than a normal vein).
D. In arterial phase of angiography, the DVA should show no AV shunting.
E. In MRI, DVAs are best visualized on T2-weighted images.

✅ The answer is **E**.
- They are best visualized on contrast-enhanced T1-weighted images.
- The "head of Medusa" is a Greek mythological figure which refers to a woman's hair that is made of serpents.
- Other angiographic descriptive terms include spokes of a wheel, an umbrella, a mushroom, or a sunburst or starburst.
- In arterial phase of angiography, the DVA should show no AV shunting (characteristic of AVM).

? 15. **DVA**
   Management, the FALSE answer is:
   A. In general, DVAs should not be treated as they are the venous drainage of the brain in that vicinity.
   B. If symptoms are present, look for an associated cavernous malformation.
   C. If surgery is indicated for associated cavernous malformations, the DVA should be left alone.
   D. Surgery for the DVA itself is reserved only for documented bleeding or for intractable seizures definitely attributed to the lesion.
   E. SRS and endovascular approach are alternative treatment options for DVAs.

✓ The answer is **E**.
   – SRS is of no benefit for venous angioma, and it is not accessible by an endovascular approach.
   – Because DVAs drain normal brain parenchyma, treatment may result in devastating venous infarcts.
   – Coexistence of a cavernoma with a venous angioma occurs in about 8 % of cases.
   – Multiple DVAs are reported to be more associated with cavernoma.

4.2   Capillary Telangiectasia

? 16. **Capillary telangiectasia (capillary malformation)**
   Pathology, the FALSE answer is:
   A. Capillary telangiectasia is a vascular malformation composed of dilated capillaries.
   B. Capillary telangiectasia contains normal intervening neural tissue.
   C. The normal intervening neural tissue is the only and the most important feature that distinguishes it from cavernomas.
   D. Microscopically, they consist of ectatic individual vessels with thin capillary walls that course among normal architectural elements.
   E. Capillary telangiectasias have adjacent gliosis or hemosiderin deposition.

✓ The answer is **E**.
   – Capillary telangiectasias are characterized by the absence of adjacent gliosis or hemosiderin deposition.

? 17. **Capillary telangiectasia**
The FALSE answer is:
   A. The most commonly detected intracranial vascular malformation in autopsy.
   B. Capillary telangiectasias are rarely symptomatic.
   C. They are most often solitary.
   D. Capillary telangiectasias are usually multiple if associated with ataxia-telangiectasia syndrome.
   E. Most commonly located in the pons.

✓ The answer is **A**.
   − Capillary telangiectasia is second most commonly detected vascular malformation in autopsy, while DVA is the most common intracranial vascular malformation in autopsy.
   − They are most often solitary; however, multiple lesions are found in sporadic or syndromic vascular malformations such as Osler-Weber-Rendu syndrome, ataxia-telangiectasia, or Wyburn-Mason syndrome.
   − Are most commonly located in the pons, but may occur elsewhere in the CNS, as well as in other organs.

? 18. **Brain capillary telangiectasia**
The FALSE answer is:
   A. The lack of a mass effect or increased T2 signal argues against other pathology.
   B. Capillary telangiectasia is a histopathological diagnosis rather than a radiologic one.
   C. Capillary telangiectasias are always diagnosed angiographically.
   D. The only vascular malformation that is composed of sacs of stagnant blood with deoxyhemoglobin.
   E. No further treatments are currently advised

✓ The answer is **C**.
   − Capillary telangiectasias are classified as "angiographically occult" lesions.
   − The only vascular malformation that is composed of sacs of stagnant blood with deoxyhemoglobin thus exhibit susceptibility dephasing, which is evident only on gradient-echo images.
   − Brain capillary telangiectasias are most often discovered in the third and fourth decades of life.
   − These lesions are usually silent on CT and angiography, but have characteristic presentations on contrast-enhanced MRI studies, specifically

demonstrating susceptibility to gradient-echo sequences and "brush"- or "stipple"-like enhancement interspersed among normal brain parenchyma. Diagnosis is based primarily on radiographic findings, and no further treatments are currently advised. Follow-up imaging may be obtained to ensure stability and to confirm the diagnosis.

4.3   Angiographically Occult (or Cryptic) Vascular Malformations (AOVMs)

19. AOVMs, not visualized due to the following factors
The FALSE answer is:
   A. Transiently occult AVMs due to destruction or compression by hematoma or edema
   B. Transiently occult AVMs due to late filling
   C. All AVMs
   D. Intraluminal thrombosis because of stagnation or sluggish flow
   E. Changes in blood vessels as spasm or dysplastic changes

✔ The answer is **C**.
   – Only micro-AVM
   – Intraluminal thrombosis because of stagnation or sluggish or turbulent flow
   – Changes in blood vessels, e.g., fibrosis, spasm, placation, or dysplastic changes

20. AOVMs
The FALSE answer is:
   A. Incidence of AOVM has been estimated as 50 % of cerebrovascular malformations.
   B. Abnormal arteriovenous connections histologically but are not revealed by catheter angiography.
   C. AOVM usually does not demonstrate mass effect or surrounding edema.
   D. The risk of hemorrhage from a cryptic vascular malformation is very low.
   E. This appears to be more common in lesions located within the posterior fossa.

✔️ The answer is **A**.
- Incidence of AOVM has been estimated as 10 % of cerebrovascular malformations.
- The risk of hemorrhage from a cryptic vascular malformation is around 0.25 % per year.
- AOVM most often may be discovered incidentally or present with seizures or headache. Less commonly they may present with progressive neurologic symptoms.

❓ 21. **AOVMs**
   The FALSE answer is:
   A. Many lesions have large patent vessels at surgery in spite of negative angiography.
   B. The presence of a histologically definable arterial component separates true occult AVMs from other occult vascular malformations.
   C. AVMs are the most common AOVM.
   D. Most of DVAs are angiographically occult.
   E. Cavernomas are most commonly an AOVM.

✔️ The answer is **D**.
- Most of DVAs are not angiographically occult.
- Many lesions have large patent vessels at surgery in spite of negative angiography, but other imaging modalities (i.e., CT, MRI) may be able to reveal these lesions.
- Mixed or unclassified angiomas account for 11 % of AOVM.

Vein of Galen Aneurysmal Malformations

This book contains some difficult questions marked with " * " sign.

© Springer International Publishing AG 2017
S.S. Hoz, *Vascular Neurosurgery*, DOI 10.1007/978-3-319-49187-5_5

❓ 1. VGAMs
   Definition, the FALSE answer is:
   A. The anatomic landmark of a VGAM is the presence of multiple arteriovenous shunts draining into a dilated median prosencephalic vein.
   B. True VGAM are mainly fed from the choroidal and other surrounding arteries.
   C. Are defined as arteriovenous fistulas in the choroid fissure supplied by the choroidal arteries and draining to the dilated median prosencephalic vein.
   D. Are defined as arteriovenous fistulas in the wall of a persistent embryonic vascular channel called the median prosencephalic vein.
   E. The median prosencephalic vein is an embryonic vessel normally present at the adult stage.

✔️ The answer is **E**.
  ▬ The median prosencephalic vein is an embryonic vessel **normally absent** at the adult stage.

❓ 2. VGAMs
   Definition, the FALSE answer is:
   A. Represent only 1 % of all cerebral vascular malformations.
   B. Represent up to 30 % of all pediatric vascular malformations.
   C. The median prosencephalic vein develops at the sixth week of gestation.
   D. The median prosencephalic vein of Markowski usually regresses during the 11th week of gestation.
   E. The vein of Galen is formed by the confluence of the internal cerebral veins only.

✔️ The answer is **E**.
  ▬ The vein of Galen is formed by the confluence of the internal cerebral veins and the basal vein of Rosenthal.
  ▬ The median prosencephalic vein of Markowski usually regresses during the 11th week of gestation, and by 3 months of gestation, the posterior part of it joins the internal cerebral veins and basal veins to form the vein of Galen.

? 3. **Vein of Galen aneurysmal malformations (VGAMs)**
   Anatomy, the FALSE answer is:
   A. The vein of Galen lies in the suprasellar cistern.
   B. The vein of Galen drains the thalamus.
   C. The vein of Galen drains the occipital lobes.
   D. The vein of Galen drains the medial temporal lobes.
   E. The vein of Galen drains the superior cerebellar vermis.

✓ The answer is **A**.
   – The vein of Galen lies in the quadrigeminal cistern.
   – The structures drained by the vein of Galen include the thalamus, the
     medial temporal lobes, the occipital lobes, and the superior cerebellar
     vermis.

? 4. **VGAMs**
   Anatomy, vein of Galen normal venous tributaries, the FALSE answer is:
   A. Veins from the ambient cistern
   B. Veins from the corpus callosum cistern
   C. Veins from the superior cerebellar cistern
   D. Veins from the sylvian cistern
   E. Veins from the velum interpositum cistern

✓ The answer is **D**.
   – The vein of Galen receives veins from the ambient, corpus callosum and
     superior cerebellar cistern, as well as the velum interpositum cistern.

? 5. **VGAMs**
   Anatomy, VGAM main arterial feeders, the FALSE answer is:
   A. The anterior choroidal arteries
   B. The posterior choroidal arteries
   C. The vertebral arteries
   D. The pericallosal arteries
   E. The thalamoperforating arteries

✓ The answer is **C**.
   – The vertebral arteries are not usual feeders for VGAM although it usually
     receives feeders from both anterior and posterior circulations.
   – True VGAM are predictably fed from the choroidal, circumferential
     mesencephalic, pericallosal, and meningeal arteries.

❓ 6. VGAMs
Yasargil classification, the FALSE answer is:
A. Type I is the most common type.
B. All types have pericallosal arteries, P3–P4 arteries, and choroidal arteries.
C. Perforators from posterior communicating arteries and P1 are absent in type I only.
D. A companion intrinsic thalamic or mesencephalic AVM is present in type IV only.
E. Internal cerebral veins, atrial vein, and mesencephalic veins are visualized on cerebral angiogram of type IV only.

✅ The answer is **A**.
  — Type III is the most common type.
  — Yasargil classified based on the arterial supply pattern of the malformation.
  — The Yasargil classification is probably the most descriptive one so far proposed, with application toward open neurosurgery, whereas the Lasjaunias system is more applicable to endovascular approaches.
  Yasargil classification of vein of Galen malformations:
  — **Type I:** Pure cisternal fistula between pericallosal arteries (anterior or posterior), posterior cerebral artery (P3–P4 and its branches), and the vein of Galen
  — **Type II:** Fistulous connections between the thalamoperforators (basilar and P1 segment) and the vein of Galen
  — **Type III:** Mixed form with characteristics of both type I and II lesions (high flow) (the most common type)
  — **Type IV:** Plexiform (parenchymal) AVM with one or more intrinsic niduses within the mesencephalon or thalamus with draining veins emptying into vein of Galen (also known as secondary type)
  — **Type IVA:** Pure plexiform nidus in the parenchyma of thalamus
  — **Type IVB:** Pure plexiform nidus in the parenchyma of mesencephalon
  — **Type IVC:** Nidus within the parenchyma combined with fistulous cisternal nidus (type I)

❓ 7. VGAMs
Lasjaunias classification, choroidal type, the FALSE answer is:
A. Choroidal type is the most common type.
B. Choroidal type is the simplest type.

C. Choroidal multiple feeders include thalamoperforating, choroidal, and pericallosal arteries.
D. The feeders are located in the subarachnoid space and the choroidal fissure.
E. The feeders converge on a fistula site at the anterior aspect of median prosencephalic vein.

✓ The answer is **B**.
▬ Choroidal type is the more complex type as compared with the mural type.

8. VGAMs
Lasjaunias classification, choroidal type, the FALSE answer is:
A. Clinically, this type is the most severe form of the disease.
B. Tend to present earlier (neonate) with more severe shunts.
C. Choroidal type results in high-output cardiac failure.
D. The multiple high-flow fistulas with less outflow restriction cause the high-output cardiac failure.
E. Lasjaunias choroidal type equals to Yasargil type I.

✓ The answer is **E**.
▬ Lasjaunias choroidal type equals to Yasargil type II.

9. VGAMs
Lasjaunias classification, mural type, the FALSE answer is:
A. Fistulae in the subarachnoid space in the wall of the median prosencephalic vein.
B. Supply may be unilateral or bilateral.
C. Associated with dilation and enlargement of dural sinuses.
D. Associated with stenosis at the level of the jugular foramen.
E. Arterial feeders arise from the collicular or quadrigeminal arteries and/ or the posterior choroidal arteries.

✓ The answer is **C**.
▬ Associated with the absence or stenosis of dural sinuses.

10. VGAMs
Lasjaunias classification, mural type, the FALSE answer is:
A. Lasjaunias mural type equals to Yasargil type I.
B. The mural type presents with fewer fistulas and high outflow restriction.

    C. The mural type is associated with stenotic and narrow median prosencephalic vein.

    D. The mural type manifests later in infancy as macrocephaly, hydrocephalus, or failure to thrive.

    E. Cardiac failure, if present, is mild and cardiomegaly may be asymptomatic.

✓ The answer is **C**.

— The mural type is associated with more severe dilation of median prosencephalic vein.

— Lasjaunias proposed an angiographic classification depending on the number and origin of feeding arteries.

Lasjaunias classification of vein of Galen malformations:

— **Choroidal type:**

    – Multiple feeders including thalamoperforating, choroidal, and pericallosal arteries are located in the subarachnoid space in the choroidal fissure.

    – Converge on a fistula site at the anterior aspect of median prosencephalic vein.

    – Tend to present earlier (neonate) with more severe shunts.

    – Clinically, this type is the most severe form of the disease.

    – This type of VGAM results in high-output cardiac failure because of multiple high-flow fistulas with less outflow restriction.

    – Type I, the choroidal type, is the most common and more complex type.

— **Mural type:**

    – Fistulae in the subarachnoid space in the wall of the median prosencephalic vein.

    – Arterial feeders arise from the collicular or quadrigeminal arteries and/or the posterior choroidal arteries.

    – Supply may be unilateral or bilateral.

    – Associated with the absence or stenosis of dural sinuses.

    – Associated with stenosis at the level of the jugular foramen.

    – This type of VGAM presents with fewer fistulas with high outflow restriction.

    – Due to the smaller number of fistulas and more outflow obstruction, they are associated with more severe dilation of the median prosencephalic vein and manifest later in infancy as macrocephaly, hydrocephalus, or failure to thrive. Cardiac failure, if present, is mild and cardiomegaly may be asymptomatic.

— New classification system proposed by Mortazavi et al.: proposed a new classification scoring system combining the previous ones and including the two most important parameters affecting outcomes reported so far: heart failure and age.

— The distinctive difference of this system is inclusion of clinical symptoms and correlation to treatment. Note exclusion of AVM and inclusion of heart failure and age as important prognostic factors.

— Mortazavi classification of vein of Galen malformations:

Score		
Parameter	**0**	**1**
Arterial feeders	Any feeders other than: P1–P2, thalamoperforators, choroidal, basilar	Any of the following feeders: P1–P2, thalamoperforators, choroidal, basilar
Symptoms	No heart failure	Heart failure
Age	≥5 months	<5 months

— Treatment related to Mortazavi classification of vein of Galen malformations:

Points	Treatment
0–1	Endovascular (no urgency); treat in 1 stage
2	Endovascular (urgency); treat in stages
3	Consider endovascular treatment or palliation; treat in stages

— Angiographic comparison of all classification systems:

Yasargil	Lasjaunias	Mortazavi
I	Type II (mural)	0
II	Type I (choroidal)	1
III		
IV (A–C)		Excluded

- Note the exclusion of true AVM in the Mortazavi classification system. Note also that there is no perfect comparison available between the three classification systems. Only the angiographic component of Mortazavi classification system is shown in this table.

? 11. **VGAMs**
Clinical feature, the FALSE answer is:
 A. Neonate presenting with almost always significant high-output cardiac failure.
 B. On examination has bulging anterior fontanelle with a bruit on auscultation.
 C. Infant presenting with hydrocephalus and/or seizures.
 D. Older child or adult presenting with headaches or SAH.
 E. The basis for most clinical symptoms is the mass effect.

✓ The answer is **E**.
- The basis for most clinical symptoms is not the mass effect, but rather the shunting of blood through the fistula that produces either cerebral or coronary artery "steal."
- Cyanosis is very common and is typically refractory to medical therapy.

? 12. **VGAMs***
Pathology, the FALSE answer is:
 A. The straight sinus is very prominent in most VGAMs.
 B. The dilated median prosencephalic vein usually drains to the embryonic falcine sinus.
 C. Embryonic falcine sinus is connected to the posterior third of the superior sagittal sinus.
 D. Persistence of other embryologic sinuses, such as the occipital and marginal sinuses, is often observed in patients with VGAMs.
 E. Persisting arterial anomalies such as a limbic arterial ring involving the anterior and posterior choroidal arteries and pericallosal arteries are also frequently present.

✓ The answer is **A**.
- The straight sinus is absent with most VGAMs.

? 13. **VGAMs***
Pathology, the FALSE answer is:
 A. Is associated with hydrodynamic disorder caused by the intracranial arteriovenous shunting.

B. The hydrodynamic disorder describes a state of disturbed absorption of CSF and venous hypertension.
C. VGMs may be associated with Down syndrome.
D. VGMs may be associated with supernumerary digits, hypospadias.
E. VGMs may be associated with transposition of great vessels, aortic stenosis, and right-sided aortic arch.

✅ The answer is **C**.
− VGMs may be associated with Turner syndrome and blue rubber bleb syndrome not Down syndrome.
− The hydrodynamic disorder describes a state of disturbed absorption of CSF and venous hypertension caused by the intracranial arteriovenous shunting that occurs in patients with VGAM.

❓ 14. VGAMs*
   Pathology (melting brain syndrome), the FALSE answer is:
   A. Melting brain syndrome describes an advanced stage of the hydrodynamic disorder.
   B. Melting brain syndrome is indicative of a poor prognosis.
   C. Cerebral blood flow is decreased because of venous hypertension, and the brain parenchyma is acutely destroyed.
   D. The ventricular system is enlarged, but intracranial pressure is not elevated.
   E. Melting brain syndrome usually occurs in adults.

✅ The answer is **E**.
− Melting brain syndrome can occur in fetuses, neonates, and infants, but it is not observed in adults.
− Cerebral blood flow is decreased because of venous hypertension, and the brain parenchyma (white matter) is acutely and progressively destroyed.
− Melting brain syndrome can be associated with all types of AV fistulas, including VGAMs, pial AVMs, and dural sinus malformations.
− Although it occurs bilaterally and symmetrically, brain atrophy around a pial AVM can be regarded as a focal expression of the same phenomenon.

❓ 15. VGAMs
   Investigations, the FALSE answer is:
   A. Mutations in the RASA 1 gene may be involved in the pathogenesis of VGAM.
   B. Contrast CT scan is the gold standard.
   C. Brain CT scan may show "ta rget sign."

    D. MRI provides greater details about the ischemic changes occurring in the affected brain.

    E. The final diagnosis of the malformation is provided by cerebral angiography.

✔ The answer is **B**.
- Cerebral angiography is the gold standard.
- CT scan shows the characteristic features, namely, calcification, low-density cystic spaces, and post-contrast enhancement.
- On CT scan, central thrombus and peripheral circulating blood along the wall of the sac can produce the so-called "target sign."
- An MRI scan is more sensitive than a CT scan since it provides better information concerning the malformation and its effects on the surrounding brain.
- An MRI scan provides greater details about the ischemic changes occurring in the affected brain and also depicts the patency and size of the large arteries, veins, and venous sinus.

❓ **16. VGAMs**
Investigations, the FALSE answer is:
    A. Prenatal ultrasonography shows the characteristic midline tubular anaechoic structure inferior to the thalamus.
    B. Prenatal ultrasonography shows "keyhole sign."
    C. Trans-fontanelle ultrasonography shows a hypoechoic midline mass with dilated lateral ventricles.
    D. Doppler evaluation is important in differentiating this lesion from other cystic lesions of the brain.
    E. VGAMs are the only lesion that clearly displays blood flow within it in Doppler evaluation.

✔ The answer is **A**.
- Prenatal ultrasonography shows the characteristic midline tubular anaechoic structure **superior** to the thalamus, which is contiguous with the dilated sagittal sinus (comet tail or keyhole sign).

❓ **17. VGAMs***
Investigations, the FALSE answer is:
    A. Differential diagnoses include arachnoid cyst and quadrigeminal cistern.
    B. Differential diagnoses include cavum vergi and cavum septum pellucidum.

C. All of the above differential show flow on Doppler evaluation.
D. Monitoring serial plasma BNP (brain natriuretic peptide) provides valuable information regarding the need for additional evaluation of newborns with CHF.
E. Serial plasma BNP is helpful as a prognostic indicator.

✓ The answer is **C**.
- Differential diagnosis includes arachnoid cyst, cavum vergi, cavum septum pellucidum, and quadrigeminal cistern. None of these show flow on Doppler evaluation, only the VAGMs show a flow.
- Monitoring serial plasma BNP provides valuable information regarding the need for additional evaluation or treatment of newborns with CHF and is also helpful as a prognostic indicator.

❓ 18. **VGAMs**
Treatment, the FALSE answer is:
A. Ideally, the initial treatment is conservative.
B. Ideally, the intervention should be delayed until the infant is 5 or 6 months old.
C. If there are clinical signs of an acute deterioration, urgent definitive treatment may be indicated.
D. The cardiac status of the patient usually improves significantly after embolization, even if complete occlusion of the VGAM cannot be achieved.
E. The radiosurgery is never used in VGAMs.

✓ The answer is **E**.
- The radiosurgery can be used and is limited to the last stage of treatment for a small residual in older children.
- Modalities may include embolization (mainstay), surgery, shunting for hydrocephalus, or a combination therapy.
- Complete occlusion of the lesion is not the objective at this age because of the increased risk for complications and limitation in the use of contrast material.
- The goal of medical treatment is to control the cardiac failure so that the baby can tolerate oral feeding and gain weight.

❓ 19. **VGAMs**
Treatment of hydrocephaly, the FALSE answer is:
A. It is best to avoid ventricular shunting.
B. The aim of the therapy is correcting the basic pathology.

   C. The results of most shunting procedures for ventriculomegaly in
      infants and neonates are excellent.
   D. If endovascular treatment is performed after the full development of
      hydrocephalus, the effect of embolization is usually insufficient.
   E. Embolization should be avoided for at least a few days after
      placement of a ventricular shunt.

✓ The answer is **C.**
   - The results of most shunting procedures for ventriculomegaly in infants
     and neonates are disappointing because intraventricular pressure is
     invariably low.
   - The aim of the therapy is correcting the basic pathology. This strategy has
     shown to normalize the head circumference.
   - If endovascular treatment is performed after the full development of
     hydrocephalus, the effect of embolization is usually insufficient, and third
     ventriculostomy or a ventricular shunt should then be considered.
   - Embolization should be avoided for at least a few days after placement of
     a ventricular shunt to avoid the risk for upward cerebellar herniation
     secondary to a rapid decrease in supratentorial pressure.
   - Although compression of the aqueduct of Sylvius by the VGAM may be
     present, obstructive hydrocephalus is rare.
   - It is also possible for the ventriculomegaly to progress without increased
     intracranial pressure because of subependymal atrophy.
   - Third ventriculostomy may be sufficient and more preferable than
     ventricular shunting for the treatment of hydrocephalus if it is combined
     with embolization of the VGAM.

❓ 20. **VGAMs**
        Treatment (indications for early intervention), the FALSE answer is:
        A. Stable cardiac failure
        B. Development of significant macrocrania or hydrocephalus
        C. Recognition of developmental delay
        D. Recognition of venous ischemic changes such as calcifications
        E. Pial venous hypertension

✓ The answer is **A.**
   - Unstable or progressive cardiac failure despite adequate medical
     treatment.
   - Chronic venous ischemia of the brain induces subcortical white matter
     calcification.

? 21. VGAMs
Yasargil classification, the FALSE answer is:
A. Embolization before or after surgery may be helpful in all types.
B. Embolization alone may be helpful in all types.
C. Microsurgery is usually reserved in medically stable patients especially for Yasargil type I.
D. Surgery is the procedure of choice for type IV.
E. Stereotactic radiosurgery is only indicated in some cases of type IV.

✔ The answer is **D**.
— Surgery is hazardous for type IV.
— Microsurgery is usually reserved in medically stable patients especially for Yasargil type I and less complex types II and III.

? 22. VGAMs*
Treatment (endovascular embolization): the FALSE answer is:
A. Transvenous embolization is the primary choice of treatment.
B. Transvenous approach is reserved for patients in whom trans-arterial embolization is impossible or unsuccessful.
C. Transvenous approach is technically easier but is associated with a higher rate of post procedure hemorrhage.
D. Transvenous approach is contraindicated when the venous pouch is connected to subependymal veins via the choroidal veins.
E. Trans-arterial embolization is most suitable for Yasargil type I, II, or III malformations.

✔ The answer is **A**.
— Trans-arterial embolization is the primary choice of treatment.
— Transvenous approach is technically easier but is associated with a higher rate of post procedure hemorrhage than is the case with trans-arterial embolization because of the sudden increase in venous back pressure with a patent fistula.
— The main complication is hemorrhage due to increased venous hypertension which can be avoided by staged procedure.

? 23. VGAMs*
Treatment (endovascular embolization), the FALSE answer is:
A. A transumbilical artery approach may be preferable in newborn.
B. For a mural-type VGAM, complete obliteration requires one or two sessions of endovascular treatment.
C. For a choroidal-type VGAM, complete obliteration requires several sessions of endovascular treatment.

     D. In most neonates, 20 ml/kg body weight of contrast material is well tolerated.

     E. The total amount of contrast material that can be tolerated by a patient depends on the duration of the procedure and urinary output.

✅ The answer is **D**.
- In most neonates, up to 8 mL/kg body weight of contrast material is well tolerated.
- A transumbilical artery approach is possible for newborn patients and sometimes preferable because of the small size of the femoral artery.
- For a mural-type VGAM, complete obliteration of the lesion can usually be achieved in one or two sessions of endovascular treatment.
- For a choroidal-type VGAM, several sessions of staged embolization may be necessary over a period of several years to achieve complete obliteration.

❓ **24. VGAMs**

Treatment (surgery), the FALSE answer is:

A. Surgery alone is the best and definitive choice for the treatment of VGAMs.

B. Microsurgery is usually reserved in medically stable patients especially for Yasargil type I.

C. Microsurgery is usually reserved in medically stable patients especially for less complex Yasargil types II and III.

D. The galenic region can surgically be approached by the subtemporal, transcallosal, or transtentorial approaches.

E. The posterior interhemispheric approach is most commonly used to adequately access a vein of Galen malformation and expose the feeding arteries.

✅ The answer is **A**.
- Surgery alone has only a limited adjunctive role for the treatment of VGAMs.
- A staged approach during the neonatal period, with the use of selective embolization or occlusion of vessels, to reduce the volume of the arteriovenous shunt until the patient is older and better able to tolerate major operation.
- Types 4A and 4B vein of Galen aneurysms carry significantly higher treatment risk for postoperative death or neurological deficit; direct intraoperative injection of thalamoperforating feeding vessels with acrylic glue can be used on these cases with some success.

❓ 25. VGAMs

Prognosis, the FALSE answer is:

A. Typically, patients with VGAMs die from a combination of cerebral and cardiac events.
B. Adults usually succumb to their cardiac insufficiency.
C. Untreated VGAMs have a poor prognosis.
D. Untreated neonates with VGAMs have nearly 100 % mortality.
E. The mortality rate is still about 35 % and significant morbidity is seen in another 30 % of patients.

✅ The answer is B.

— Neonates usually succumb to their cardiac insufficiency, while older children and adults usually succumb to the cerebral injury.
— Untreated VGAMs have a poor prognosis, with neonates having nearly 100 % mortality, and 1–12 month olds having 60 % mortality, 7 % major morbidity, and 21 % being normal.

❓ 26. VGAMs*

Lasjaunias (Bicêtre) neonatal scoring system, the FALSE answer is:

A. Lasjaunias have described a 21-point scale based on cardiac, cerebral, hepatic, respiratory, and renal functions.
B. A score of less than 8 usually indicates a good prognosis.
C. A score of less than 8 usually does not warrant emergency management.
D. A score of 8–12 is an indication for emergency endovascular management.
E. A score of more than 12 indicates a well-preserved neonate, and attempts are made to delay the endovascular procedure, by medical management.

✅ The answer is B.

— A score of less than 8 usually indicates a poor prognosis.

Bicêtre neonatal evaluation score					
Points	Cardiac function	Cerebral function	Respiratory function	Hepatic function	Renal function
5	Normal	Normal	Normal	-	-
4	Overload, no medical treatment	Subclinical, isolated EEG abnormalities	Tachypnea, finishes bottle	-	-

Bicêtre neonatal evaluation score					
Points	Cardiac function	Cerebral function	Respiratory function	Hepatic function	Renal function
3	Failure, stable with medical treatment	Nonconvulsive intermittent neurologic signs	Tachypnea, does not finish bottle	No hepatomegaly, normal hepatic function	Normal
2	Failure, not stable with medical treatment	Isolated convulsion	Assisted ventilation, normal saturation FIO2 < 25 %	Hepatomegaly, normal hepatic function	Transient anuria
1	Ventilation necessary	Seizures	Assisted ventilation, normal saturation FIO2 > 25 %	Moderate or transient hepatic insufficiency	Unstable diuresis with treatment
0	Resistant to medical therapy	Permanent neurological signs	Assisted ventilation, desaturation	Abnormal coagulation, elevated enzymes	Anuria

- EEG (electroencephalogram), FIO2 (fractional inspired oxygen)
- Maximal score: 21 (5 cardiac, 5 cerebral, 5 respiratory, 3 hepatic, 3 renal)

? 27. VGAMS*

Other types, the FALSE answer is:

A. Vein of Galen Varix indicates dilation of vein of Galen without the presence of an AV shunt.

B. Vein of Galen aneurysmal dilation in contrast to VGAM: the midline ectatic vein in this group is the true vein of Galen, and it therefore receives drainage from the normal brain, as well as the malformation.

C. Pial AVMs with vein of Galen aneurysmal dilation, usually initially manifested in childhood or young adulthood as intracerebral hemorrhage, focal neurological deficit, or seizures.

D. Dural AVMs with vein of Galen aneurysmal dilation is an acquired lesion in which AV shunts are located in the wall of the vein of Galen itself.

E. Endovascular treatment is easy and of choice for dural AVMs with vein of Galen aneurysmal dilation.

✅ The answer is **E**.
- Dural arteriovenous malformation with vein of Galen aneurysmal dilation: endovascular treatment of this type of dural AVM had been difficult because the transvenous approach is often not feasible and there are too many feeders from both the carotid and vertebral arteries for trans-arterial embolization.
- Dural AVMs with vein of Galen aneurysmal dilation is an acquired lesion in which AV shunts are located in the wall of the vein of Galen itself; typical clinical findings are headaches and progressive dementia.
- Vein of Galen Varix: VGV indicates dilation of the vein of Galen without the presence of an AV shunt and it is usually asymptomatic.
- Vein of Galen Varix: Two types have been encountered in children. One is transient asymptomatic dilation of the vein of Galen in neonates with cardiac failure from a cause other than VGAM. This dilation is usually noticed on an ultrasound study and disappears in several days after improvement of the cardiac condition. The second type of VGV occurs as an anatomic variation in which venous drainage of the brain converges toward the deep venous system. It is also asymptomatic, but this arrangement of venous drainage may predispose to future venous thrombosis and resultant ischemic symptoms because of the lack of compliance.
- Pial arteriovenous malformation with vein of Galen aneurysmal dilation: For treatment, transvenous occlusion of the venous dilation in the VGAD is contraindicated because it may produce hemorrhage or venous infarction of the deep cerebral structures as a result of occlusion of the outflow of these veins. Demonstration of trans-mesencephalic feeders by magnetic resonance imaging (MRI) or angiography confirms the pial nature of the lesion.

Moyamoya Disease

This book contains some difficult questions marked with " * " sign.

© Springer International Publishing AG 2017
S.S. Hoz, *Vascular Neurosurgery*, DOI 10.1007/978-3-319-49187-5_6

❓ 1. Moyamoya Disease (MMD)
Definition, the FALSE answer is:

A. A rare chronic cerebrovascular disease characterized by stenosis-occlusion of the bilateral ICAs at their terminal portion and subsequent development of peculiar moyamoya vasculature at the base of the brain.
B. The term moyamoya means "something hazy, like a puff of smoke."
C. The term moyamoya describes the characteristic angiographic appearance of abnormally dilated collateral vessels in MMD.
D. An increasingly recognized cause of stroke.
E. MMD is the most common pediatric cerebrovascular disease worldwide.

✔ The answer is **E.**
- MMD including 6 % of all strokes in children.
- In Japan, it is the most common pediatric cerebrovascular disease.
- Rare chronic cerebrovascular disease characterized by stenosis-occlusion of the bilateral ICAs at their terminal portion (carotid fork) and the subsequent development of peculiar moyamoya vasculature at the base of the brain.
- The term moyamoya comes from a Japanese expression for something "hazy just like a puff of cigarette smoke drifting in the air" was first described by Suzuki and Takaku in 1969.

❓ 2. MMD
Definition, the FALSE answer is:

A. To have moyamoya disease, patients usually have bilateral stenosis.
B. Patients with only unilateral findings have moyamoya syndrome.
C. Individuals with a well-recognized associated condition are categorized as having moyamoya syndrome.
D. Idiopathic cases with no known risk factors have moyamoya syndrome.
E. The term moyamoya, when used alone without the modifier of disease or syndrome, refers to the distinctive findings on arteriography, independent of etiology.

✔ The answer is **D.**
- Individuals with a well-recognized associated condition are categorized as having moyamoya syndrome, whereas idiopathic cases with no known risk factors have moyamoya disease.

Classification of moyamoya
Moyamoya disease:
- Bilateral, idiopathic steno-occlusive supraclinoid carotid disease
- Bimodal age of diagnosis: 5 and 40 years old
- Predominantly Asian heritage
- Twice as common in females as in males

Moyamoya syndrome:
- Associated disease state
- Unilateral carotid disease (even if idiopathic)
- Variable epidemiology

Atypical moyamoya:
- Moyamoya vessels in non-carotid distribution
- Associated aneurysm or pseudoaneurysms
- Associated arteriovenous malformation

❓ 3. **MMD**
Definition, the FALSE answer is:
A. A bimodal age distribution of moyamoya, one group in the pediatric age range and a second group of adults in the 30- to 40-year-old range.
B. Moyamoya affects young children in particular, with 50 % of patients identified by 10 years of age.
C. Males are affected nearly twice as often as females.
D. Asian Americans are more than four times as likely to have moyamoya.
E. African Americans are twice as likely to have moyamoya.

✔️ The answer is **C**.
- Females are affected nearly twice as often as males.
- Its incidence is higher in Asian countries than in Europe or North America.
- Asian Americans are more than four times as likely, African Americans are twice as likely, and Hispanic Americans are half as likely to have moyamoya.

❓ 4. **MMD**
Pathology, the FALSE answer is:
A. In all cases, the process extends to involve the posterior circulation.
B. The proximal portion of the PCA is also involved in around half of affected patients.
C. Pathologic analysis has demonstrated that affected vessels generally do not exhibit arteriosclerotic or inflammatory changes.

D. Pathologic analysis has demonstrated that vessel occlusion results from a combination of both hyperplasia of smooth muscle cells and luminal thrombosis.

E. Occlusion of the anterior circulation occurs simultaneously as characteristic arterial collateral vessels develop at the base of the brain in response to the resultant ischemia.

✅ The answer is **A**.
- Rarely, in advanced cases, the process can extend to involve the posterior circulation, including the basilar artery and PCA.

❓ 5. **MMD**
Pathology, the FALSE answer is:
A. The moyamoya collaterals are dilated perforating arteries believed to be a combination of preexisting and newly developed vessels.
B. The familial incidence of affected first-degree relatives is 7–12 %.
C. Basal moyamoya have abnormally dilated collaterals via the dural arteries.
D. Ethmoidal moyamoya have abnormally dilated collaterals via the ethmoidal arteries.
E. Vault moyamoya have abnormally dilated collaterals via the dural arteries.

✅ The answer is **C**.
- MMD is also characterized by an extensive peculiar development of collateral pathways: (1) **basal moyamoya** in the basal ganglia and thalamus, namely, abnormally dilated collaterals via the lenticulostriate arteries, the anterior choroidal artery, the posterior choroidal artery, and the posterior communicating artery, (2) **ethmoidal moyamoya** via the anterior and posterior ethmoidal arteries originating from the ophthalmic artery, and (3) **vault moyamoya** via the dural arteries, also called transdural anastomosis.

❓ 6. **MMD**
Pathology, the FALSE answer is:
A. The moyamoya vessels are thin walled, with a paucity of smooth muscle cells and incomplete internal elastic lamina.
B. The moyamoya vessels never have aneurysmal dilatations.
C. It is from the moyamoya (abnormal) vessels that the risk of ICH, IVH, and SAH arises.

D. The ECA collateral networks providing extracranial (EC)-to-intracranial (IC) anastomoses also develop.
E. The EC-to-IC anastomoses particularly from middle meningeal, ethmoidal, and occipital arteries.

✅ The answer is **B**.
- The moyamoya vessels may harbor aneurysmal dilatations.
- The moyamoya vessels show increased expression of growth factors.

❓ **7. MMD, association, the FALSE answer is:**
A. Moyamoya is strongly associated with radiotherapy for gliomas.
B. Moyamoya is strongly associated with radiotherapy for pituitary tumors.
C. Moyamoya is associated with Down syndrome.
D. Moyamoya is strongly associated with neurofibromatosis type II.
E. Moyamoya is associated with sickle cell anemia.

✅ The answer is **D**.
- Strong associations exist between moyamoya and radiotherapy of the head or neck (especially for optic gliomas, craniopharyngiomas, and pituitary tumors), Down syndrome, **neurofibromatosis type I** (with or without hypothalamic-optic pathway tumors), and sickle cell anemia.

❓ **8. MMD***
   Genetics, the FALSE answer is:
A. Moyamoya may be associated with mutation in loci on chromosomes 3.
B. Moyamoya may be associated with mutation in loci on chromosomes 6.
C. Moyamoya may be associated with mutation in loci on chromosomes 8.
D. Moyamoya may be associated with specific HLA haplotypes.
E. Moyamoya is strongly associated with haplotype at chromosome 2.

✅ The answer is **E**.
- Associations between moyamoya and loci on chromosomes 3, 6, 8, and 17 (MYMY1, MYMY2, MYMY3), as well as specific HLA haplotypes, have been described.
- A single haplotype of the RNF213 locus at chromosome **17q** is strongly associated with moyamoya disease. Mutation analysis of RNF213 identified a founder mutation present in 95 % of Japanese familial moyamoya disease, 73 % of nonfamilial moyamoya disease, and only 1.4 % of controls.

? 9. **MMD**

Presentation, the FALSE answer is:
A. Cerebral ischemic events are more common in children.
B. Cerebral hemorrhages are more common in Asian adults.
C. Cerebral ischemic events are more common in white adults.
D. Cerebral hemorrhages are more common in males.
E. Cerebral ischemia is the next most common manifestation in adults.

✓ The answer is **D.**
— Intracranial bleeding is the typical finding in Asian adults, especially females (up to 66 %).
— The clinical findings are mainly cerebral ischemia in children and cerebral hemorrhage in Asian adults, but presumably also mainly ischemia in white adults.
— TIAs is the most common finding (70 % to 80 %) in children.
— The clinical features of moyamoya result from either direct cerebral ischemia (e.g., stroke, TIA) or the deleterious effects of responses to this ischemia (e.g., hemorrhage from fragile collateral vessels, headache as a result of dural irritation from collaterals).

? 10. **MMD**

Presentation, the FALSE answer is:
A. The symptoms of cerebral ischemia in moyamoya are generally related to the territory supplied by the ICAs.
B. The watershed areas at the border zones between arterial territories are particularly susceptible.
C. Hemiparesis, dysarthria, aphasia, and cognitive impairment are common.
D. TIAs are common in children who are not precipitated by hyperventilation.
E. Seizures occur frequently.

✓ The answer is **D.**
— TIAs may be precipitated by events particularly common in children, such as hyperventilation with crying or exertion.
— The symptoms of cerebral ischemia in moyamoya are generally related to the territory supplied by the ICAs, including the frontal and temporal lobes.

- The cerebral vessels, already maximally dilated in the setting of chronic ischemia, constrict in response to the decrease in PCO_2 and can thus lead to a TIA or stroke.
- Dehydration, a problem in children after colds or fevers, may also give rise to ischemic symptoms.

? 11. MMD
Presentation, the FALSE answer is:
   A. Typically, hemorrhage is a hallmark of adult moyamoya, although children can also have this finding initially.
   B. Hemorrhage can be IVH, ICH, or rarely SAH.
   C. Children with moyamoya will often complain of headache.
   D. Headache often completely relieved after surgery before other symptoms remit.
   E. Collateral vessels in the basal ganglia have also been implicated in the development of choreiform movements in individuals with advanced moyamoya.

The answer is D.
- Children with moyamoya will often complain of headache. Although it may improve after surgical treatment of the moyamoya, often concordant with regression of the collateral vessels, it often persists as troublesome symptom years after other symptoms remit.
- Hemorrhage can be IVH, ICH (frequently in the region of the basal ganglia), or rarely SAH.
- Similar to headache, choreiform movements may regress after revascularization of the affected hemisphere.

? 12. MMD
Presentation, the FALSE answer is:
   A. Bleeding has historically been attributed to rupture of fragile collateral vessels unable to contain the increased flow shunted from progressive ICA stenosis.
   B. Rebleeding carries an even graver prognosis.
   C. Rebleeding is often occurring at the same original bleeding site.
   D. Rupture of microaneurysms in the periventricular region can cause intracranial bleeding.
   E. Fibrinoid necrosis of the arterial wall in the basal ganglia causes intracranial bleeding.

✅ The answer is **C**.
- Rebleeding is often occurring at a location different from the original bleeding site.
- There are three main causes of intracranial bleeding in patients with MMD: (1) rupture of dilated and stressed perforating arteries containing microaneurysms, (2) fibrinoid necrosis of the arterial wall in the basal ganglia, and (3) rupture of microaneurysms in the periventricular region, especially around the superolateral wall of the lateral ventricles.

❓ 13. **MMD and associated aneurysms**
The FALSE answer is:
  A. Saccular cerebral aneurysms, a possible cause of a rather rare SAH in this disease.
  B. Saccular cerebral aneurysms occur mainly around the circle of Willis.
  C. Saccular cerebral aneurysms can occur in the abnormal moyamoya vasculature.
  D. These false aneurysms will never disappear spontaneously.
  E. These false aneurysms might need to be removed surgically because of repeated bleeding.

✅ The answer is **D**.
- These false aneurysms may disappear spontaneously or after revascularization procedures.
- Saccular cerebral aneurysms are detected in 4–14 % of patients, and 16 % of these patients have been reported to have multiple aneurysms.
- These aneurysms occur in three locations: (1) 60 % around the circle of Willis, mainly at the vertebro-basilar territory; (2) 20 % in peripheral arteries, such as the posterior and anterior choroidal arteries; and (3) 20 % in the abnormal moyamoya vasculature.

❓ 14. **MMD**
Natural history, the FALSE answer is:
  A. Any child with new symptoms of cerebral ischemia should be considered as a possible moyamoya patient until prove otherwise.
  B. The rate of disease progression is high even in asymptomatic patients.
  C. Two-thirds of patients with moyamoya have symptomatic progression.

D. Patients with moyamoya have poor outcomes if left untreated.

E. Age of the patient predicts long-term outcome more than neurological status at time of treatment.

✓ The answer is **E**.

– Neurological status at time of treatment, more so than age of the patient, predicts long-term outcome.

❓ **15. MMD**

Radiology, the FALSE answer is:

A. Hemorrhage or small areas of hypo-density in CT scan suggestive of stroke are commonly observed in the cortical watershed zones, basal ganglia, deep white matter, or periventricular regions.

B. T1-weighted MRI is sensitive in detecting basal moyamoya.

C. Chronic infarction is best seen with diffusion-weighted imaging.

D. Diminished cortical blood flow secondary to moyamoya can be inferred from FLAIR sequences, which demonstrate the so called "ivy sign."

E. The "ivy sign" is a leptomeningeal high-signal intensity along the cortical sulci seen on FLAIR or contrast-enhanced T1-weighted sequences in MMD.

✓ The answer is **C**.

– Acute infarction is best seen with diffusion-weighted imaging.

– Chronic infarction is better demonstrated on T1- and T2-weighted MRI.

– Leptomeningeal high-signal intensity along the cortical sulci may be seen on FLAIR or contrast-enhanced T1-weighted sequences in moyamoya disease patients. This is referred to as the **ivy sign** and is thought to reflect slow flow in cortical vessels. Differential diagnosis: leptomeningeal metastases, hemorrhage, meningitis, and high oxygen tension or hyperbaric O_2 (100 % O_2).

❓ **16. MMD**

Radiology, the FALSE answer is:

A. Cerebral angiography is presently mandatory for definitive diagnosis, even if MRI and MRA clearly fulfill the criteria.

B. Cerebral angiography has a solid position in the management of MMD, especially in the planning for surgery.

C. Cerebral angiography is important for postoperative evaluation.

D. The diagnosis of MMD is defined by angiography and is characterized by bilateral stenosis of the distal intracranial ICA extending to the proximal ACA, MCA, and PCA.

E. Reduced flow voids in the ICA, MCA, and ACA coupled with prominent flow voids from the basal ganglia and thalamic collateral vessels are considered to be essentially diagnostic of moyamoya.

✅ The answer is **A**.
- Cerebral angiography is presently not necessary for definitive diagnosis if MRI and MRA clearly fulfill the criteria.

❓ **17. MMD**
Radiology, the FALSE answer is:

A. Cerebral angiography has been emphasized in the diagnostic criteria for MMD known as the six-stage classification.

B. The first three stages are narrowing of the carotid fork, initiation of the moyamoya, and intensification of the moyamoya.

C. The next three stages are minimization of the moyamoya, reduction of the moyamoya, and disappearance of the moyamoya.

D. Stage IV is the least frequently encountered.

E. Stage II includes "initiation of the moyamoya."

✅ The answer is **D**.
Stage IV is encountered most frequently.

Moyamoya staging (Suzuki):[1]
Stage I
- "Narrowing of the carotid fork"
- Narrowed ICA bifurcation

Stage II
- "Initiation of the moyamoya"
- Dilated ACA, MCA, and narrowed ICA bifurcation with moyamoya change

Stage III
- "Intensification of the moyamoya"
- Further increase in moyamoya change of the ICA bifurcation and narrowed ACA and MCA

Stage IV
- "Minimization of the moyamoya"
- Moyamoya change reducing with occlusive changes in ICA and tenuous ACA and MCA

---

[1] Descriptions in inverted commas are those of Suzuki in the original paper.

Stage V
- "Reduction of the moyamoya"
- Further decrease in moyamoya change with occlusion of ICA, ACA, and MCA

Stage VI
- "Disappearance of the moyamoya"
- ICA essentially disappeared with supply of the brain from ECA

Diagnostic criteria of moyamoya disease:

A. Cerebral angiography is indispensable for diagnosis and should show at least the following findings:
   1. Stenosis or occlusion at terminal portion of the ICA and/or at proximal portion of ACAs and/or MCAs
   2. Abnormal vascular networks in the vicinity of the occlusive or stenotic lesions in arterial phase
   3. Findings should appear bilaterally

B. When MRI and MRA demonstrate all subsequently described findings, conventional cerebral angiography is not mandatory:
   1. Stenosis or occlusion at terminal portion of ICA and at the proximal portion of ACAs and MCAs on MRA.
   2. An abnormal vascular network in the basal ganglia on MRA. An abnormal vascular network can be diagnosed when more than two apparent flow voids are observed in one side of the basal ganglia on MRI.
   3. (1) and (2) are observed bilaterally.

C. Because the origin of this disease is unknown, cerebrovascular disease with the following basic diseases or conditions should be eliminated:
   1. Arteriosclerosis
   2. Autoimmune disease
   3. Meningitis
   4. Brain neoplasm
   5. Down syndrome
   6. Recklinghausen disease
   7. Head trauma
   8. Irradiation to the head
   9. Others (e.g., sickle cell disease, tuberous sclerosis)

D. Instructive pathological findings:
1. Intimal thickening and resulting stenosis or occlusion of lumen observed in and around terminal portion of ICA, usually on both sides. Lipid deposits occasionally noted in proliferating intima.
2. Arteries constituting the circle of Willis such as the ACAs, MCAs, and posterior communicating arteries often show stenosis of various degrees or occlusion associated with fibrocellular thickening of intima, waving of the internal elastic lamina, and attenuation of media.
3. Numerous small vascular channels (perforators and anastomotic branches) observed around circle of Willis.
4. Reticular conglomerates of small vessels often noted in pia mater.

Diagnosis: In reference to A to D, the diagnostic criteria are classified as follows (autopsy cases not undergoing cerebral angiography should be investigated separately while referring to D):
1. Definite case: Fulfills criteria A or B and C. Pediatric case that fulfills A-1 and A-2 (or B-1 and B-2) on one side. Remarkable stenosis at terminal portion of ICA on opposite side also included.
2. Probable case: Fulfills criteria A-1 and A-2 (or B-1 and B-2) and C (unilateral involvement).

❓ 18. MMD*
Radiology, the FALSE answer is:
A. EEG and cerebral blood flow studies may be helpful in the evaluation.
B. Specific findings on EEG are usually found in pediatric patients.
C. The induced hyperventilation for EEG is highly recommended in a patient with known moyamoya.
D. Cerebral blood flow studies include techniques such as transcranial Doppler.
E. Cerebral blood flow studies can help quantify blood flow.

✅ The answer is **C.**
— The induced hyperventilation for EEG is **not** recommended in a patient with known moyamoya.
— Specific findings on EEG, usually in pediatric patients, include posterior or centro-temporal slowing, a hyperventilation-induced diffuse pattern of monophasic slow waves (i.e., buildup), and a characteristic "rebuildup" phenomenon.

- Cerebral blood flow studies include techniques such as transcranial Doppler, perfusion CT, xenon-enhanced CT, PET, MR perfusion imaging, and SPECT with acetazolamide challenge.
- Cerebral blood flow studies can help quantify blood flow, information that may be incorporated into treatment algorithms for children with moyamoya.

? 19. MMD
   Medical treatment, the FALSE answer is:
   A. Medical therapy has occasionally been used for the treatment of moyamoya.
   B. Antiplatelet agents have been administered routinely in majority patients.
   C. Calcium channel blockers are never used.
   D. Anticoagulants such as warfarin are rarely used.
   E. Phenylephrine is used during and after induction of anesthesia to prevent even transient hypotension.

✓ The answer is **C.**
- Calcium channel blockers are **useful** in ameliorating the symptoms of intractable headache or migraine, commonly seen in moyamoya patients.
- Current treatments are designed to prevent strokes by improving blood flow to the affected cerebral hemisphere, not to reverse the primary disease process.
- Reduction of ischemia can protect against future strokes, effect a concurrent reduction in the number and size of collateral vessels, and improve symptoms, but it does not arrest the underlying carotid arteriopathy.

? 20. MMD
   Surgery, the FALSE answer is:
   A. Indirect revascularization is without microvascular anastomotic procedures.
   B. Indirect bypass is often technically difficult to perform in adults.
   C. Direct revascularization combined with an indirect procedure is considered to be the therapy of choice in adults.
   D. Direct revascularization can selectively perfuse ischemic areas immediately.
   E. Direct revascularization can cause hyperperfusion syndrome as a complication.

✓ The answer is **B**.
- Direct bypass is often technically difficult to perform in **children** because of the small size of donor and recipient vessels.
- Prompt treatment should be done once moyamoya is identified.
- Two surgical methods are used: direct and indirect.
- Direct revascularization is done via microvascular extracranial-to-intracranial bypass, while indirect revascularization is without microvascular anastomotic procedures.
- The indirect technique is more appealing in pediatric populations.
- Direct revascularization techniques or combining them with an indirect procedure is considered to be the therapy of choice in adults because indirect methods alone have been reported to be unpredictable or ineffective in achieving good revascularization.
- Direct revascularization can selectively perfuse ischemic areas immediately but, in so doing, may cause hyperperfusion syndrome as a complication.
- Although indirect revascularization techniques, employing onlay synangiosis, have proven very successful in the pediatric population, direct revascularization with bypass (alone or in combination with onlay techniques) may offer more benefit for adult patients.

? 21. **MMD**
Surgery (indirect bypass techniques) includes, the FALSE answer is:
A. Encephalo-duro-arterio-myo-synangiosis (EDAMS).
B. Encephalo-myo-synangiosis (EMS).
C. Simply drilling bur holes without vessel synangiosis.
D. Occipital artery-PCA bypass.
E. A modification termed pial synangiosis has been used with encouraging results in both adults and children.

✓ The answer is **D**.
- Occipital artery-PCA bypass is a direct bypass technique.

? 22. **MMD**
Surgery (indirect bypass techniques) includes, the FALSE answer is:
A. Indirect techniques involve mobilizing vascularized tissue and placing it in contact with the brain.
B. EMS facilitates gradual revascularization according to the needs of the ischemic brain.
C. Protection from ischemia is usually immediate.

    D. EDAMS is the preferred technique for indirect revascularization.
    E. EMS is used in the absence of an appropriate cortical branch of the MCA on the surface of the brain.

✅ The answer is **C**.
- Protection from ischemia is delayed for several weeks with indirect techniques while new vessel ingrowth is established.
- Indirect techniques involve mobilizing vascularized tissue supplied by the ECA and placing it in contact with the brain to facilitate ingrowth of new vessels to the cortex.
- One reason for EMS use may be the infrequent existence of an appropriate cortical branch of the MCA on the surface of the brain in patients with MMD, especially children, which makes direct revascularization difficult or impossible.

❓ 23. **MMD**
    Surgery (indirect bypass donor sites) include, the FALSE answer is:
    A. The inverted convexity dura
    B. The superficial temporal vein
    C. The vascularized pericranium
    D. The temporalis muscle
    E. The omentum

✅ The answer is **B**.
- Non-vessel donor tissues for indirect revascularization include the fascial cuff surrounding the STA, the inverted convexity dura, the vascularized pericranium, the temporalis muscle, and the omentum.

❓ 24. **MMD***
    Surgery (direct bypass techniques), the FALSE answer is:
    A. Adults with a remarkable drop in performance could benefit from an STA-ACA bypass.
    B. Patients with visual disturbances could benefit from an STA-PCA bypass.
    C. In occipital artery-PCA bypass, the trunk of the PCA must be occluded.
    D. In occipital artery-PCA bypass, the recipient artery is the posterior temporal branch of PCA.
    E. Occipital artery-PCA bypass can be done by supracerebellar transtentorial approach.

✔️ The answer is **C.**

- Performance of the occipital artery-PCA bypass via the supracerebellar transtentorial approach in the sitting position has the advantage that the trunk of the PCA **does not need to be temporarily occluded** for the anastomotic procedure; the posterior temporal artery, which courses over the parahippocampal gyrus at its posterior portion, is used as a recipient artery.
- Adults with a remarkable drop in performance because of low perfusion in the ACA territory could benefit from an STA-ACA bypass in combination with a standard STA-MCA bypass.
- In patients with low perfusion of the PCA territory and visual disturbances, an STA-PCA or occipital artery-PCA bypass may be considered.

❓ 25. MMD*

Surgery, the FALSE answer is:

A. Surgery is performed when the hemodynamic and metabolic situation has stabilized.
B. Patient with frequent ischemic episodes should undergo urgent surgery.
C. If any significant changes on EEG occur as the initial side is operated on, surgery on the contralateral hemisphere is postponed.
D. Any techniques to reduce pain may reduce the likelihood of stroke.
E. Avoid the use of hyperventilation.

✔️ The answer is **B.**

- Surgery should be scheduled during a period when the patient is in a relatively stable clinical condition **without** frequent ischemic episodes.
- Sufficient hydration should be ensured.
- Preoperative evaluation of hemodynamic dysfunction with acetazolamide loading should be carried out with caution.
- Without these careful measures, serious ischemic complications have been reported to occur at rates of up to 10 % or greater.
- Avoid the use of hyperventilation or any anesthetic technique that would cause cerebral vasoconstriction. Crying and hyperventilation can lower $PaCO_2$ and induce ischemia secondary to cerebral vasoconstriction.
- Any techniques to reduce pain (perioperative sedation, painless wound dressing, and closure with absorbable suture) may reduce the likelihood of stroke and shorten the hospitalization.

? 26. MMD*
Surgery (direct bypass techniques), the FALSE answer is:
A. Donor vessels for revascularization are most commonly the STA.
B. Donor vessels include MMA or occipital artery.
C. STA arises from the ECA within the substance of the parotid gland.
D. The recipient vessel for bypass is usually an M2 branch of the MCA.
E. Common branches used in direct technique are the angular, posterior temporal, and posterior parietal arteries.

✓ The answer is **D**.
- The recipient vessel for bypass is usually an M4 branch of the MCA, which begins as the vessel exits the sylvian fissure and courses over the cortical surface.
- The STA is one of the two terminal branches of the ECA. It arises from the ECA within the substance of the parotid gland, courses over the posterior root of the zygomatic process of the temporal bone, and divides into a frontal branch that runs anterosuperiorly and a parietal branch that runs superiorly in the subgaleal plane of the scalp.
- Donor vessels for revascularization include the frontal or parietal branches of the STA or, less commonly, the middle meningeal artery (MMA) and the occipital artery.

? 27. MMD
Outcome, the FALSE answer is:
A. Bilateral involvement eventually develops in approximately a third of patients with unilateral moyamoya.
B. Mortality in the acute stage with the infarction type is higher than the hemorrhagic type.
C. The progression of the disease is more likely to occur rapidly in younger patients.
D. The progression of the disease is more frequently in younger patients.
E. The annual risk for any stroke in these patients is around 3 %.

✓ The answer is **B**.
- Mortality in the acute stage has been reported to be low: 2.4 % with the infarction type and 16.4 % with the hemorrhagic type.
- Patients with unilateral MMD should be monitored carefully because 7–27 % of such patients, including children, have been reported to progress to bilateral disease within a few years of follow-up.
- The annual risk for any stroke in these patients has been reported to be 3.2 %.

? 28. MMD*

Outcome, the FALSE answer is:

A. The majority of cases have a benign course in terms of life expectancy, with or without surgical treatment.

B. After revascularization procedures, the majority of adult patients with MMD are free of TIAs and ischemic strokes.

C. Rebleeding occurs in about 30–65 % of patients during follow-up.

D. Pregnancy and delivery may increase the risk for ischemic or hemorrhagic stroke in female patients.

E. Angiography 1 year postoperatively and then no further follow-up is needed.

✓ The answer is **E**.

- Follow-up is by angiography for 1 year postoperatively and then annual MRI studies for several years thereafter.
- 75–80 % of cases are thought to have a benign course in terms of life expectancy, with or without surgical treatment.
- Many institutions perform angiography 1 year postoperatively, followed by annual MRI studies for several years thereafter.

Spinal Vascular Malformations

This book contains some difficult questions marked with " * " sign.

© Springer International Publishing AG 2017
S.S. Hoz, *Vascular Neurosurgery*, DOI 10.1007/978-3-319-49187-5_7

❓ 1. Spinal arteriovenous malformations (SAVM)
Incidence, the FALSE answer is:
   A. Incidence of SAVM is about 4 % of primary intraspinal masses.
   B. It represents one-tenth of the brain AVMs.
   C. SAVM shows a male predominance.
   D. SAVM usually extends over a single segment.
   E. SAVM usually presents in the fourth or fifth decade.

✅ The answer is **D.**
   ▬ SAVM usually extends over four or five segments, and as a rule they are located posterior or posterolateral in the caudal spinal canal.

❓ 2. SAVM
Diagnosis, the FALSE answer is:
   A. The most common presentation for SAVM is progressive neurological deficit.
   B. The diagnostic modality of choice for SAVM is spinal angiography.
   C. CT scan findings are usually normal unless SAH.
   D. The MRI usually localizes the exact fistula site.
   E. Digital subtraction arteriography is the criterion standard modality for visualizing SAVM in real time.

✅ The answer is **D.**
   ▬ The MRI, in particular, allows visualization of thrombosed veins and of the spinal cord, but the exact fistula site **cannot be** localized.
   ▬ The most common presentation for SAVM is progressive neurological deficit (subacute to chronic onset of back pain, weakness, sensory loss).
   ▬ Spinal angiography: necessary to confirm the diagnosis and to identify major feeding vessels, this might be suitable for embolization and for treatment planning.
   ▬ Digital subtraction arteriography allowing the assessment of high-flow versus low-flow AVMs, in addition, the location of the fistula can be visualized.

❓ 3. SAVM
Types, the FALSE answer is:
   A. Type I is dural AVF.
   B. Type II is intramedullary or glomus AVM.
   C. Type II is the most common type.
   D. Type III is juvenile or combined AVMs.
   E. Type IV is perimedullary AVF.

✅ The answer is **C**.
- Type I is the most common type.
- Anson and Spetzler classification (1992) is most widely used.
- A recently proposed classification of spinal cord vascular lesions has added extradural AVFs and conus medullaris AVMs as distinct entities.

❓ 4. **SAVM**
Types, the FALSE answer is:
A. Type I is high flow, fed by radicular arteries.
B. Type II is high flow fed by medullary arteries.
C. Type III is intraparenchymal, high flow.
D. Type III is an enlarged form of type II that invades the entire cross section of the cord.
E. Type IV: perimedullary, often fed by the artery of Adamkiewicz and the anterior spinal artery.

✅ The answer is **A**.
- Type I: **low flow** (most common type, fed by radicular arteries)
- Type II: intraparenchymal, high flow (fed by medullary arteries)
- Type III: intraparenchymal, high flow (an enlarged form of type II that invades the entire cross section of the cord as well as the vertebral body)
- Type IV: perimedullary (often fed by the artery of Adamkiewicz and the anterior spinal artery)

❓ 5. **SAVM**
Type I, the FALSE answer is:
A. The most common type of malformation comprises 80–85 % of SAVM.
B. These lesions are most frequently found in females.
C. Usually presented between the fifth and eighth decades of their life.
D. Is dural/intradural dorsal AVFs.
E. A dural AVF that arises at the dural nerve root sleeve.

✅ The answer is **B**.
- These lesions are most frequently found in males (90 % are males).
- Type 1: They are also known as intradural dorsal AVFs, angiomas racemosum, angioma racemosum venosum, long dorsal AVFs and dorsal extramedullary AVFs.

? 6. SAVM

Type I, the FALSE answer is:

A. Is fed by radicular artery which forms an AV shunt located in the intervertebral foramen
B. Drains into an engorged spinal vein on posterior cord
C. Most occur spontaneously
D. May be of acquired etiology
E. Direct communication between an extradural artery and extradural vein with nidus

✓ The answer is **E.**

— Direct communication between an extradural artery and extradural vein with no nidus
— Is fed by radicular artery which forms an AV shunt (fistula) at the dural root sleeve (located in the intervertebral foramen)

? 7. SAVM

Type I, the FALSE answer is:

A. They are predominantly found in the posterior part of the lower thoracic cord and the conus.
B. They may be found in the conus.
C. Dural AVFs are predominantly located on the right side.
D. Type IA has single arterial feeder.
E. Type IB has two or more arterial feeders.

✓ The answer is **C.**

— Dural AVFs are predominantly located on the left side.
— For type I dural AVMs, angiography must encompass all dural feeders of the neuraxis, which includes:
— ICAs include the artery of Bernasconi and Cassinari
— Every radicular artery including the artery of Adamkiewicz
— Internal iliac arteries: for sacral feeders

? 8. SAVM

Type I, the FALSE answer is:

A. 15–20 % is associated with other AVMs (cutaneous or other).
B. Patients become symptomatic because of the venous congestion and hypertension of the spinal cord.
C. The absence of valves between the coronal and radicular veins decreases the venous congestion.

    D. Presented as gradual progressive radiculomyelopathy.

    E. Presented rarely as acute presentation and rarely bleed.

✅ The answer is **C**.
- The absence of valves between the coronal and radicular veins encourages venous congestion.
- Patients with dural AVFs become symptomatic because the AVF creates venous congestion and hypertension resulting in hypoperfusion of the spinal cord.

❓ **9. SAVM**
    Type I, the FALSE answer is:
    A. Symptoms tend to be exacerbated by Valsalva maneuvers.
    B. Foix-Alajouanine syndrome: chronic neurologic deficit in a patient with a spinal AVM without evidence of hemorrhage.
    C. Foix-Alajouanine syndrome is due to venous thrombosis from spinal venous stasis.
    D. Coup de poignard of Michon: onset of SAH with sudden excruciating back pain.
    E. Gadolinium MRI has proven useful in revealing the level of the fistula before angiography.

✅ The answer is **B**.
- Foix-Alajouanine syndrome: **acute or subacute neurologic deterioration** in a patient with a spinal AVM without evidence of hemorrhage.
- Foix-Alajouanine syndrome is an extreme form of spinal dural AVF that affects a minority of patients who present with a rapidly progressive myelopathy due to venous thrombosis from spinal venous stasis.
- Coup de poignard of Michon: onset of SAH with sudden excruciating back pain (clinical evidence of Spinal AVM).
- Gadolinium MRI has proven useful in revealing the level of the fistula before angiography. Angiography helps in treatment planning of the fistula.

❓ **10. SAVM**
    Type I, the FALSE answer is:
    A. The recommended treatment is surgery or embolization.
    B. Dural AVFs can be treated with either open or endovascular ligation usually with poor results.

   C. Open surgery is necessary if the arterial feeding vessel is impossible to access.
   D. Open surgery is necessary if the feeding vessel supplies healthy regions of the spinal cord.
   E. Exposure of the fistula may be achieved by hemilaminectomy.

✅ The answer is **B**.
  ▬ Dural AVFs can be treated with either open or endovascular ligation with excellent results.
  ▬ Open surgery is necessary if the arterial feeding vessel is impossible to access because of tortuous vascular anatomy or if the vessel supplies blood to healthy regions of the spinal cord.

❓ 11. **SAVM**
   Type I, the FALSE answer is:
   A. Coagulation of abnormal vascular structures on the dural layer may be done.
   B. Excision of the whole area of abnormality.
   C. Ligation and section at the site of the fistula without stripping the dilated veins that drain the normal spinal cord is recommended.
   D. Stripping may precipitate clinical deterioration.
   E. Surgery has shown to have a high rate of recurrence.

✅ The answer is **E**.
  ▬ Surgery has shown to have a low rate of recurrence or persistent fistula.
  ▬ Coagulation of abnormal vascular structures on the dural layer or excision of the whole area of abnormality or both may be done.

❓ 12. **SAVM**
   Type II, the FALSE answer is:
   A. Is the true AVM of the spinal cord
   B. Is an intramedullary AVMs or glomus AVMs
   C. Constitute 15–20 % of all SVMs
   D. Multiple feeders from the anterior and posterior spinal artery
   E. Low-flow and high-resistance drainage into medullary veins

✅ The answer is **E**.
  ▬ High-flow and low-resistance drainage into medullary veins located in the anterior half of the cord with intramedullary nidus.

? 13. SAVM
   Type II, the FALSE answer is:
   A. Compact nidus fed by medullary arteries with the AV shunt contained at least partially within the spinal cord or pia.
   B. Fed by one or at most two to three feeders in 80 % of the time.
   C. In contrast to dural AVFs, glomus AVM arises in a younger population and is believed to be of congenital origin.
   D. They are typically located in the anterior half of the cord.
   E. They are more common in the sacral region.

✓ The answer is **E.**
   — They are more common in the cervical region

? 14. SAVM
   Type II, the FALSE answer is:
   A. The lesion may be compact or diffuse.
   B. The lesion may contain groups of intramedullary arterial and venous vessels (nidus) inside a short segment of the spinal cord.
   C. Associated arterial or venous aneurysm may be present in most of cases.
   D. Presented as progressive and fluctuating myelopathy.
   E. Often overlaid by periods of acute neurologic deterioration secondary to hemorrhage within the AVM.

✓ The answer is **C.**
   — Associated arterial or venous aneurysm may be present in 20–40 % of cases.
   — The lesion may be compact or diffuse with groups of intramedullary arterial and venous vessels (nidus) inside a short segment of the spinal cord.
   — Often overlaid by periods of acute neurologic deterioration secondary to hemorrhage within the AVM.

? 15. SAVM
   Type II, the FALSE answer is:
   A. They can present with mass effect caused by growth of the AVM, impairing neurologic function.
   B. The SAH with sudden apoplectic presentation is very rare.
   C. The SAH often with profound neurologic impairment.
   D. After initial hemorrhage, the rebleed rate is 10 % within the first month.
   E. After initial hemorrhage, the rebleed rate is 40 % within the first year.

✔ The answer is **B**.
- The SAH with sudden apoplectic presentation is common.
- The SAH often with profound neurologic impairment secondary to their location, which is usually the dorsal cervicomedullary region.

❓ **16.   SAVM**
   Type II, the FALSE answer is:
   A. Spinal AVM should be considered in the differential diagnosis of any patient with a SAH who has negative cerebral angiography results.
   B. Acute nonhemorrhagic deterioration may be related to other pathology.
   C. In MRI, a localized dilatation of the spinal cord can be demonstrated because of the intramedullary location.
   D. The feeding and draining vessels appear as low-signal, round, long, and serpiginous structures.
   E. The lesion may be surrounded by hemosiderin ring.

✔ The answer is **B**.
- Acute nonhemorrhagic deterioration may be related to spontaneous venous thrombosis.
- The feeding and draining vessels appear as low-signal, round, long, and serpiginous structures surrounded by areas of low signal on T1- and T2-weighted images due to hemosiderin of previous hemorrhages.

❓ **17.   SAVM**
   Type II, the FALSE answer is:
   A. Because these lesions often compromise the anterior spinal artery, a definitive cure is usually obtained with surgery.
   B. Surgery for compact ones with or without embolization and embolization alone for diffuse ones.
   C. Compact nidus is most amenable to surgical resection through a standard myelotomy between the two posterior columns.
   D. Has better prognosis than dural AVM.

✔ The answer is **E**.
- Has worse prognosis than dural AVM.
- Embolizing major feeders is helpful during surgery.

❷ 18. SAVM
   Type III, the FALSE answer is:
   A. Known as juvenile AVMs.
   B. Also known as combined intramedullary and extramedullary AVMs.
   C. Essentially an enlarged glomus AVM which occupies the entire cross section of the cord.
   D. Usually invades the vertebral body which may cause scoliosis.
   E. Tiny low-flow AVM of the spinal cord parenchyma fed by multiple intramedullary and extramedullary vessels.

✅ The answer is **E**.
   ▬ Large high-flow AVM of the spinal cord parenchyma fed by multiple intramedullary and extramedullary vessels.
   ▬ Essentially an enlarged glomus AVM which occupies the entire cross section of the cord and invades the vertebral body which may cause scoliosis.

❷ 19. SAVM
   Type III, the FALSE answer is:
   A. Progressive and fluctuating myelopathy with acute presentation is extremely rare.
   B. Auscultatable spinal bruit may be present.
   C. They can involve several levels.
   D. They may be intramedullary and extramedullary in location.
   E. They may involve the skin, muscle, bone, and spinal cord.

✅ The answer is **A**.
   ▬ Progressive and fluctuating myelopathy with acute presentation is not uncommon.
   ▬ They usually involve the entire metamere compromising the skin, muscle, bone, and spinal cord (this manifestation is known as Cobb's syndrome).

❷ 20. SAVM
   Type III, the FALSE answer is:
   A. They occur most commonly in adolescents and young adults.
   B. Presentation and treatment are similar to that of glomus type.
   C. Treatment is largely considered palliative, multidisciplinary, and multistage.
   D. Radiosurgery may be considered.
   E. Prognosis for these lesions is good with high rate of cure.

✅ The answer is **E**.
 — A multidisciplinary and multistaged treatment is recommended.
 — Prognosis for these lesions, considering their size and vascular complexity, is understandably **very poor**, although reports of improvement and occasional case reports of cure do exist.

❓ **21. SAVM**
 Type IV, the FALSE answer is:
 A. Type IV is a perimedullary AVFs.
 B. Type IV is an arteriovenous fistula.
 C. Fistula is between anterior spinal artery (often artery of Adamkiewicz) and a spinal vein with no nidus.
 D. Located dorsal to the spinal cord.
 E. They are mostly found at the thoracic level.

✅ The answer is **D**.
 — **TYPES IV SAVM** is located ventral to the spinal cord.
 — Type IV is an intradural perimedullary AVM (also called arteriovenous fistula AVF).

❓ **22. SAVM**
 Type IV, the FALSE answer is:
 A. Type IV is present in the third to sixth decade.
 B. Typically occur in younger patients than type I.
 C. Acute presentation is common.
 D. Type IV has a female predominance.
 E. A gradual progressive myelopathy is due to arterial steal and resultant ischemia.

✅ The answer is **C**.
 — Acute presentation is uncommon.
 — May present catastrophically with SAH.
 — A gradual progressive myelopathy (due to arterial steal and resultant ischemia) is common.

❓ **23. SAVM**
 Type IV subcategory, the FALSE answer is:
 A. Type IVc is the most common type of type IV SAVM.
 B. Type IVa has multiple giant fistulas.
 C. Type IVa and IVb have slow ascending venous drainage.

D. Type IVc is the only one with single arterial supply of type IV SAVM.

E. Type IVc has single giant fistula.

✅ The answer is **B**.

━ Type IVa has **single small** fistula.

━ Three subcategories are described with Anson and Spetzler's nomenclature of a, b, and c.

━ **Type IV**: intradural perimedullary (AV fistula)

  ━ **Type IVa:**

  – Single arterial supply (ASA)

  – Single small fistula

  – Slow ascending perimedullary venous drainage

  ━ **Type IVb:**

  – Multiple arterial supply (ASA and PSA)

  – Multiple medium fistulas

  – Slow ascending perimedullary venous drainage

  ━ **Type IVc:**

  – Multiple arterial supply (ASA and PSA)

  – Single giant fistula

  – Large ectatic venous drainage

❓ **24. SAVM***

Type IV subcategory, the FALSE answer is:

A. Type IVa, surgical excision is often required.

B. Type IVa, endovascular techniques are difficult due to the small size of feeding vessels.

C. Type IVb, embolization is more difficult due to the small size of feeding vessels.

D. In cases of incomplete shunt obliteration with an endovascular approach, direct surgical excision may be necessary.

E. Type IVc, spinal ischemia may develop in these lesions secondary to vascular steal.

F. Type IVc, treatment is through combination of endovascular ablation, followed by surgical excision of retained elements.

✅ The answer is **C**.

━ Type IVb, embolization is easier due to the increased size of feeding vessels.

━ Type IVa, features a single feeding vessel, often the artery of Adamkiewicz, with low flow through the arteriovenous shunt and moderate venous enlargement. Endovascular techniques are difficult with these lesions due to the small size of feeding vessels. Surgical excision is therefore often required.

- Type IVb arteriovenous fistulas are intermediate in size, often with multiple feeding vessels and more marked venous enlargement. Venous ectasia may develop at the site of shunting. Embolization in these lesions is easier due to the increased size of feeding vessels. In cases of incomplete shunt obliteration with an endovascular approach, direct surgical excision may be necessary.
- Type IVc features giant, multipediculated fistulas, high blood flow, and large tortuous draining veins. Spinal ischemia may develop in these lesions secondary to vascular steal. Treatment is through combination of endovascular ablation, followed by surgical excision of retained elements. Due to the size of these lesions, surgery is technically difficult and may jeopardize the spinal cord. Good outcomes usually follow endovascular treatment. If endovascular treatment is unsuccessful, the fistula can be interrupted surgically.

25. SAVM*
Conus AVMs, the FALSE answer is:
A. Conus AVMs are recently added entity to spinal AVMs.
B. Conus AVMs are characterized by both an anterior and dorsal intradural AVF.
C. Conus AVMs are characterized by multiple feeders and an intramedullary AVM.
D. An abnormality during neurulation has been proposed to explain their development.
E. Patients with conus AVM usually present with radicular symptoms only.

The answer is **E.**
- Patients with conus AVM usually present with myelopathy or radicular symptoms.

26. SAVM*
Conus AVMs, the FALSE answer is:
A. Early bowel and bladder compromise reflects their typical location at the conus.
B. Cono-caudal presentation is rare.

    C. Their extensive nature and multiple arterial feeders make it difficult to treat.

    D. It is difficult to treat conus AVMs by embolization alone.

    E. An initial embolization followed by surgical resection is ideal.

✅ The answer is **B**.
- Cono-caudal presentation is likely.

❓ **27. Spinal cavernoma**
   The FALSE answer is:
   A. Spinal cavernomas constitute 5 % of spinal vascular malformations.
   B. Spinal cavernomas constitute 5 % of all CNS cavernomas.
   C. Patients with spinal cavernomas rarely harbor intracranial cavernoma, so brain MRI is rarely indicated.
   D. Spinal cavernomas managed essentially the same as brainstem cavernomas and complete excision is mandatory.
   E. In spinal cavernomas, if symptoms recur after surgery in the absence of residual cavernomas, a tethered cord should be considered.

✅ The answer is **C**.
- 42 % of patients with spinal cavernomas also harbor one intracranial cavernoma, so brain MRI is mandatory.
- Spinal cavernomas are managed essentially the same as brainstem cavernomas, and complete excision is mandatory because of high risk of hemorrhage recurrence.
- Spinal cavernomas usually intramedullary (superficial) location. Extradural lesions more vascular and are formidable surgical challenges because of hemorrhage. Dorsal or exophytic lesions are easier to treat.

❓ **28. Spinal aneurysms***
   The FALSE answer is:
   A. Spinal aneurysms are extremely rare.
   B. The diagnosis should be considered when no other sources of bleeding are found.
   C. The diagnosis should be considered when the SAH is limited to the spine.
   D. Aneurysms seldom occur at branching points unlike intracranial ones.
   E. Partial thrombosis of spinal aneurysms, render all of them to be asymptomatic.

✅ The answer is **E**.
- Partial thrombosis of spinal aneurysms, a frequent finding during surgery, probably accounts for their becoming **symptomatic**.
- The spinal arteries are much smaller than that of intracranial arteries, and they tend to be less affected by atherosclerosis.

❓ 29. **Spinal aneurysms***
The FALSE answer is:
  A. On MRI, they appear as round, well-localized flow voids within the spinal canal.
  B. Spinal aneurysms lack a clear neck and usually appear as fusiform dilations.
  C. Spinal aneurysms are amenable for clipping.
  D. If the aneurysm is distal on the circulation or thrombosed, the parent vessel can be occluded and the aneurysm can be removed.
  E. Endovascular techniques can be considered.

✅ The answer is **C**.
- Spinal aneurysms are **not** amenable for clipping.
- Wrapping may be considered if there is evidence of flow distal to the aneurysm; surgical reconstruction with a terminoterminal anastomosis is an option.

Service Part

© Springer International Publishing AG 2017
S.S. Hoz, *Vascular Neurosurgery*, DOI 10.1007/978-3-319-49187-5

Suggested Reading

Abdulrauf SI. Cerebral revascularization. Philadelphia: Elsevier/Saunders; 2011.

Alexander M, Spetzler R. Pediatric neurovascular disease. New York: Thieme; 2006.

Butler P. Endovascular Neurosurgery. London: Springer London; 2000.

Byrne J. Tutorials in endovascular neurosurgery and interventional neuroradiology. Berlin: Springer; 2012.

Cho B, Tominaga T. Moyamoya disease update. Tokyo: Springer; 2010.

Deshaies EM, Eddleman CS, Boulos AS. Handbook of neuroendovascular surgery. New York: Thieme; 2012.

Ellenbogen RG, Abdulrauf SI, Sekhar LN. Principles of neurological surgery. Philadelphia: Saunders/Elsevier; 2012.

Forsting M, Cognard C. Intracranial vascular malformations and aneurysms. Berlin: Springer; 2006.

Fox J. Intracranial aneurysms. Springer: New York; 1983.

Gasco J. The essential neurosurgery companion. New York: Thieme; 2013.

Gonzalez LF, Albuquerque FC, McDougall CG. Neurointerventional techniques. 2015.

Greenberg MS, Greenberg MS. Handbook of neurosurgery. Tampa: Greenberg Graphics; 2016.

Harbaugh R et al. Neurosurgery knowledge update. Thieme; 2015.

Harrigan M, Deveikis J. Handbook of cerebrovascular disease and neurointerventional technique. Totowa: Humana/Springer; 2009.

Jabbour PM. Neurovascular Surgical Techniques. New Delhi: Jaypee Brothers Medical Publishers (P) Ltd; 2013.

Kobayashi S, Goel A, Hongo K. Neurosurgery of complex tumors and vascular lesions. New York: Churchill Livingstone; 1997.

Koos WT, Spetzler RF, Lang J. Color atlas of microneurosurgery. Stuttgart [etc.]: Georg Thieme; 1997. Volume 2: Cerebrovascular Lesions.

Laakso A. Surgical management of cerebrovascular disease. Wien: Springer-Verlag; 2010.

Lanzino G, Spetzler R. Cavernous malformations of the brain and spinal cord. New York: Thieme; 2008.

Lasjaunias P. Vascular diseases in neonates, infants and children. Berlin: Springer; 1997.

Lawton M. Seven aneurysms. New York: Thieme; 2011.

Lawton M, Probst K. Seven AVMs. Thieme; 2014.

Macdonald R. Neurosurgical operative atlas. New York: Thieme; 2009.

Mitsos A. Endovascular neurosurgery through clinical cases. Milano: Springer; 2015.

Nader R et al. Neurosurgery tricks of the trade. Cranial. New York: Thieme; 2014.

Nussbaum E, Mocco J. Cerebral revascularization. New York: Thieme; 2011.

Osborn AG. Osborn's Brain. Salt Lake City: Amirsys Pub; 2013.

Radiopaedia.org

Rinkel GP. Subarachnoid hemorrhage in clinical practice. Cham: Springer; 2015.

Schmidek & sweet operative neurosurgical techniques. 2012.

Sekhar LN. Atlas of neurosurgical techniques-brain. New York: Thieme; 2015.

Sindou M. Practical handbook of neurosurgery. Wien: Springer-Verlag; 2009.

Spetzler RF, Kalani Y, Nakaji P. Neurovascular surgery. Thieme; 2015.

Steiger H. Neurosurgery of arteriovenous malformations and fistulas. Wien: Springer; 2002.

Steiger H, Etminan N, Hänggi D. Microsurgical brain aneurysms. Berlin: Springer; 2015.

Stieger PE, Batjer HH, Samson DS. Intracranial arteriovenous malformations. New York: Informa Healthcare; 2007.

Tandon PN, Ramamurthi R. Ramamurthi and tandon's textbook of neurosurgery. New Delhi: Jaypee Brothers Medical Publishers; 2012.

Tsukahara T. Trends in neurovascular surgery. Vienna: SpringerWienNew York; 2011.

Veznedaroglu E. Controversies in vascular neurosurgery: Springer; 2016.

Vincent AT. Textbook of contemporary neurosurgery. New Delhi: Jaypee Brothers Medical Publisher Pvt. Ltd; 2012.

Wanebo J, Khan N, Zabramski J, Spetzler R. Moyamoya disease. New York: Thieme; 2014.

Yaşargil MG. Microneurosurgery. Stuttgart: Thieme; 1994. Volumes: 1, 2 and 3.

Yonekawa Y. Changing aspects in stroke surgery. Wein: Springer; 2008.

Youmans J, Winn H. Youmans neurological surgery. Philadelphia: Elsevier/Saunders; 2011.

Index

GPSR Compliance

The European Union's (EU) General Product Safety Regulation (GPSR) is a set of rules that requires consumer products to be safe and our obligations to ensure this.

If you have any concerns about our products, you can contact us on ProductSafety@springernature.com

In case Publisher is established outside the EU, the EU authorized representative is:

Springer Nature Customer Service Center GmbH
Europaplatz 3
69115 Heidelberg, Germany

Batch number: 09635429

Printed by Printforce, the Netherlands